LAW AND ETHICS
IN THE
MEDICAL OFFICE

Including Bioethical Issues

LAW AND ETHICS IN THE MEDICAL OFFICE

Including Bioethical Issues

MARCIA A. LEWIS, RN, M.A., CMA-C
Instructor, Medical Assisting
Olympic College
Bremerton, Washington

CAROL D. WARDEN, B.S., CMA-A
Program Director, Medical Assisting
Highline Community College
Seattle, Washington

Foreword by Jeffrey P. Smith, Legal Counsel
Washington State Medical Association

F.A. DAVIS COMPANY 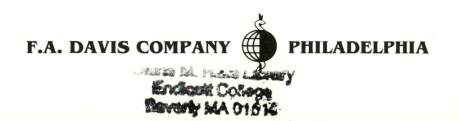 **PHILADELPHIA**

Library of Congress Cataloging in Publication Data

Lewis, Marcia A.
  Law and ethics in the medical office.

  Includes index.
    1. Medical laws and legislation—United States.
2. Medical ethics—United States. I. Warden,
Carol D. II. Title. [DNLM: 1. Allied health
personnel. 2. Ethics, Medical. 3. Legislation,
Medical. W 32.6 L675L]
KF3821.L48 1983   344.73′041   82-9993
ISBN 0-8036-5616-5   347.30441

FOREWORD

Law and Ethics in the Medical Office for the first time sets forth in a clear and concise manner the legal and ethical requirements that *all* medical office employees must meet. Each chapter outlines problems that arise everyday in the medical office and suggests methods of dealing with the problems or refers the reader to an appropriate resource. The authors have provided both students and medical office personnel with an excellent reference that I hope you will use to provide quality, compassionate health care to your patients.

Jeffrey P. Smith
Legal Counsel
Washington State Medical Association

PREFACE

This book was created to provide an adequate resource in the study of medical law and ethics for the medical office employee. While much is written on both subjects, little is oriented toward the medical office setting. It is recognized that usually the first contact a patient has with the physician is through the office employee—medical assistant, receptionist, secretary, clinical assistant, or office nurse—when the first telephone call is made or the patient steps through the front door.

It is imperative that the medical office employee has a knowledge of the law, medical ethics, and bioethics so that the patient may be treated with understanding, sensitivity, and compassion. No matter what the medical office employee's education and experience may be, any direct patient contact requires ethical and legal responsibility. It is also imperative that this knowledge be used to provide the best possible service for the physician-employer.

This book describes the laws pertinent to the office setting, outlines various ethical codes and their current impact on society, and discusses major ethical issues in medicine today.

Each chapter is preceded by learning objectives designed for the educational setting. The discussion questions are intended to be thought-provoking rather than a test of chapter contents. References are provided for anyone seeking additional information.

The authors' hope is that you will derive from this book a great sense of pride in and responsibility for your important profession as a medical office employee.

MAL
CDW

ACKNOWLEDGMENTS

It is never possible to fully acknowledge all persons who make contributions to the writers of a book. The effort requires assistance from too many individuals and sources. We wish to thank, however, a few who were especially helpful. Without them, the book would have been impossible.

Robert G. Martone, Allied Health Editor of F. A. Davis Company/Publishers, realized the book's potential and continually encouraged us throughout the process.

Jeffrey P. Smith, Legal Counsel, Washington State Medical Association, provided essential legal advice for each chapter and has written the Foreword.

Support staff included three eager and excellent typists who helped make our deadline. These friends are Shirley Baumgart, Marjorie Pierson, and Hazel West.

E. Curtiss Pierson, Managing Editor of the *Spokane Daily Chronicle* and personal friend, graciously reviewed the entire manuscript.

Students in our classes helped identify the need for this book and participated in the field testing of the manuscript. Their comments have influenced the final product.

The support of families was an essential ingredient from the inception of the book to its completion. Les, Martiann, and Steve Lewis and Jay, Jayne, and Duuana Warden shared totally in this experience. They provided encouragement where we were discouraged, and cheered when we were successful.

Thanks Marti! Thanks Carol!

MAL
CDW

CONTENTS

CHAPTER 1

INTRODUCTION TO LAW

LEARNING OBJECTIVES

Upon successful completion of this chapter, you will:

1. Explain in a brief paragraph why knowledge of the law is necessary for medical office employees.

2. Describe, using an outline, the four sources of law.

3. List the three branches of government in the United States.

4. Define:
   a. constitutional law
   b. common law
   c. statutory law
   d. administrative law
   e. plaintiff
   f. defendant
   g. felony
   h. misdemeanor.

5. List two similarities and dissimilarities between:
   a. criminal and civil law.

6. Review, in diagram form, the process for a:
   a. civil case
   b. misdemeanor case
   c. felony case.

continues on next page

7. Diagram:
   a. Federal Court system
   b. State Court system.
8. List two factors that determine in which court a case is heard.
9. Explain in your own words the trial process.

DEFINITIONS

Appellant. One who appeals a court decision to a higher court.

Arraignment. The procedure of calling someone before a court to answer a charged offense.

Civil Case. Court action between private parties, corporations, government bodies, or other organizations; compensation usually monetary; recovery of private rights.

Closing Arguments. Summary and last statements made by opposing attorneys at a hearing or trial.

Court of Appeals. Court that reviews decisions made by a lower court; may reverse, remand, modify, or affirm lower court decision. No live testimony.

Criminal Case. Court action brought by the state against individual(s) or groups of people accused of committing a crime; punishment usually imprisonment and/or a fine; recovery of rights of society.

Cross Examination. Examination of witness(es) by opposing attorney at a hearing or trial.

Defendant. The person or group accused in a court action.

Direct Examination. Examination of witness(es) by the attorney calling the witness at a hearing or trial.

Examination of Witness(es). Questioning of witness(es) by attorneys during a court action.

Felony. A serious crime such as murder, larceny, assault, rape; punishment usually severe.

Higher or Superior Court: A court with broader judicial authority than a lower or inferior court.

Judge. A public official who directs court proceedings, instructs the jury on the law governing the case, and pronounces sentence.

Jury. Six to twelve individuals, usually randomly selected, who are administered an oath to serve through court proceedings to reach a fair verdict based on the evidence presented.

Law. Rule or regulation that is advisable or obligatory to observe.

Litigation. A law suit; a contest in court.

Lower or Inferior Court. A court with limited judicial authority.

Misdemeanor. A type of crime less serious than a felony.

Opening Statement(s). Statements made by opposing attorneys at the beginning of a court action to outline what they hope to establish in the trial.

Plaintiff. The person or group initiating the action in litigation.

Probate Court. State court that handles wills and settles estates.

Sentencing. Imposition of punishment in a criminal proceeding.

Small Claims Court. Special court intended to simplify and expedite the handling of small claims or debts.

Verdict. Findings or decision of a jury on a matter submitted to it in trial.

INTRODUCTION

One cannot be employed in a medical office very long without becoming aware of the law and its impact on the activities therein. Laws are man-made rules or regulations that are advisable or obligatory to observe. Such a mandate is worthy of further discussion.

Laws have governed mankind and the practice of medicine for thousands of years. Today there are laws in all states regulating medical practice. A brief look at these laws, their sources, and their definitions is important for further discussion.

SOURCES OF LAW

Law encompasses rules derived from several sources. The Constitution of the United States provides the highest judicial authority in the United States. Adopted in 1787, it provides the framework for our government. The *Constitution*, Federal law, and treaties take precedence over the constitutional law of the states.

The United States Constitution is a legal document that defines the structure and function of Federal, state, and local governments. The Federal government has three branches: (1) *Legislative*—the lawmaking body, that is, Congress; (2) *Executive*—administrator of the law, that is, the President; (3) *Judicial*—judge or courts, that is, the Supreme Court. Each branch provides a system of checks and balances for the other two. For example, the power of lawmaking belongs to Congress, but the President can veto its legislation. The Judiciary is empowered to review the legislations. Congress, in turn, can investigate the President and control the appeal jurisdiction of the Federal courts. No one branch is a divine or absolute authority. In addition, each state has a constitution defining its own specific governing bodies. All powers not conferred upon the Federal government are retained by the state. Yet states vary widely in their execution of that power.

Many of the legal doctrines applied by the courts in the United States are products of the *common law* developed in England. This is a body of law based on judicial decisions that attempts to apply general principles to the specific situations that may arise. Common law, also called judge-made law, is as binding as constitutional law.

As society grew more complex, these common laws were not sufficient. Legislative bodies were then formed and their enactments became known as *legislative or statutory law*. These laws make up the bulk of our laws as they exist today. Publications containing these statutes are known as "codes." An example pertaining to the medical office is Medical Practice Acts, which define and outline the practice of medicine in a given state.

Legislative bodies, however, do not have the time or knowledge to enact all laws necessary for the smooth functioning of the government. Thus, administrative agencies were given the power to enact regulations that also have the force of law and are called *administrative law*. The Internal Revenue Service and Federal Trade Commission are examples of administrative agencies.

Administrative law impacts the medical office employee. The state health department, the state board of medical examiners, and the state board of nurse examiners are administrative agencies that dictate rules and regulations for the medical office. Further, licensing and accrediting bodies, as well as government programs such as Medicare and Medicaid, directly influence many policies, procedures, and functions of the medical office.

CIVIL / CRIMINAL LAW

Law is often more recognized by its classification than its source. These main classifications are civil, criminal, international, and military. The latter two are not considered here. Civil and criminal law, however, are considered because of their importance in the medical office setting.

Civil law was developed from Roman law. Civil law is a "civil code" system adopted by the legislature. It is fundamentally a collection of basic principles to be applied to individual cases. Louisiana is the only state that retains a modified civil law.[1] Civil law affects regulations between individuals. Restitution for a civil wrong is usually monetary in nature. The bulk of law dealt with in the medical office is civil in nature.

Criminal law involves laws pertaining to crimes and punishment of persons violating the law. Criminal law affects relations between individuals and the government. Criminal wrongs are acts against the welfare and safety of the public or society as a whole. Punishment for criminal acts is usually imprisonment and/or a fine.

To illustrate civil and criminal law, consider the following situation. Drunk driver Bill is involved in an automobile accident responsible for the death of a 35-year-old homemaker with two small children. Bill is charged by law enforcement with driving while intoxicated, speeding, and recklessness. The courts later find Bill guilty. This is *criminal law* protecting society. Taking this situation a step further, consider the following events:

The husband of the 35-year-old homemaker sues Bill for a substantial monetary amount to care for the two small children now without a mother. Based upon the facts of the case, the court grants an agreed-upon amount. This is *civil law*.

LEGAL SYSTEMS

Our legal system may seem complex but there is some logic to the development and existence of courts and their jurisdiction.

TYPES OF CASES

All legal matters filed in courts are classified as civil or criminal. *Civil cases* are disputes between private parties, corporations, government bodies, or other organizations. The restitution is usually monetary. In the medical office, most legal actions are of a civil nature.

In a *civil case* the party bringing the action (plaintiff) must prove the case by presenting the evidence that is more convincing to the judge or jury than the opposing evidence. Consider, for example, a "slip, trip, and fall" case. Fran enters her physician's office, slips, and falls as she approaches the reception desk. She suffers a simple fracture of the left femur. When the receptionist comes to her aid, Fran discovers a snag from the rug that caught the heel of her shoe. Fran later takes civil action and sues her physician for medical fees and loss of employment. As the plaintiff, she must prove that her physician (defendant) was negligent and she did not contribute to her injury.

The procedure for a civil case is shown in Figure 1. The plaintiff's complaint is filed in the proper court, usually by an attorney for the plaintiff. The defendant is formally summoned, prepares an answer, and files it in the court. If the defendant fails to answer the summons within the prescribed time, the plaintiff will win the case by default and judgment will be entered against the defendant.

The case may be settled without a trial; for example, the complaint may be dismissed due to some technical error, the summons may have

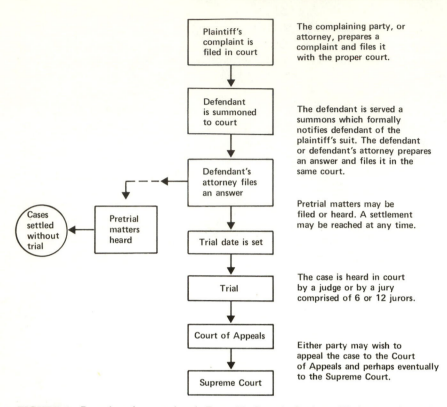

FIGURE 1. Procedure for a civil trial. From "A Citizen's Guide to Washington Courts," prepared by the Washington State Office of Administrator for the Courts to assist the public in understanding the judicial system in that state. Check for similar brochures in your state.

been improperly served, the case may not set forth a claim recognized by law, or the parties may decide to settle out of court.

If, however, the defendant's attorney files an answer, and no problems occur, the trial date is set. A case is heard in a court by a judge or jury, which makes a decision. Once a verdict is given and the judgment is rendered, either party may wish to appeal to the Court of Appeals and perhaps eventually to the Supreme Court.

Criminal cases, on the other hand, are brought by the state against individuals or groups of people accused of committing a crime. The prosecuting, district, or state's attorney prosecutes the charge against the accused person (defendant) on behalf of the state (plaintiff). The crime is an act against society. The prosecution must prove that the defendant is guilty beyond a reasonable doubt. In other words, the prosecution must be able to prove to the satisfaction of the court that a criminal act was, in fact, committed by the accused.

The crimes are normally of two types, felonies and misdemeanors. They are statutorily defined and created. Felonies are more serious crimes and include murder, larceny (thefts of large amounts of money), assault, and rape. Gross misdemeanors or misdemeanors are considered lesser offenses. These include disorderly conduct, thefts of small amounts of property, and breaking into an automobile.

Betty, Dr. G's bookkeeper, is disgruntled that her employment has been terminated and she is being replaced by a new employee. She takes a costly briefcase-sized minicomputer from the doctor's desk. Knowing it will be missed, she decides it can be blamed on the custodian. She further rationalizes that the doctor owes her that much. This is an example of a felony. Both the misdemeanor and felony case processes are shown in Figures 2 and 3, respectively.

The procedure for a misdemeanor case is shown in Figure 2. The prosecuting attorney is made aware of violations of the law in four ways, by traffic or police citations, by police arrest, or by citizen information. When enough evidence is present, the court arraigns the person. The charged

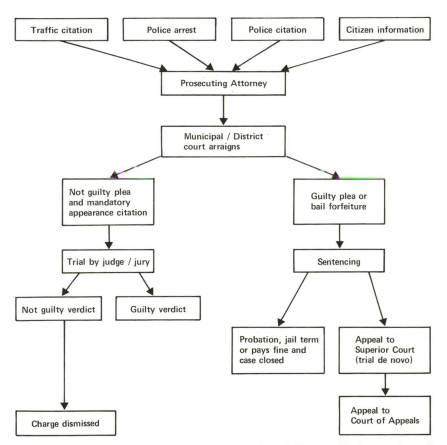

FIGURE 2. Misdemeanor case process. From "A Citizen's Guide to Washington Courts," Washington State Office of Administrator for the Courts.

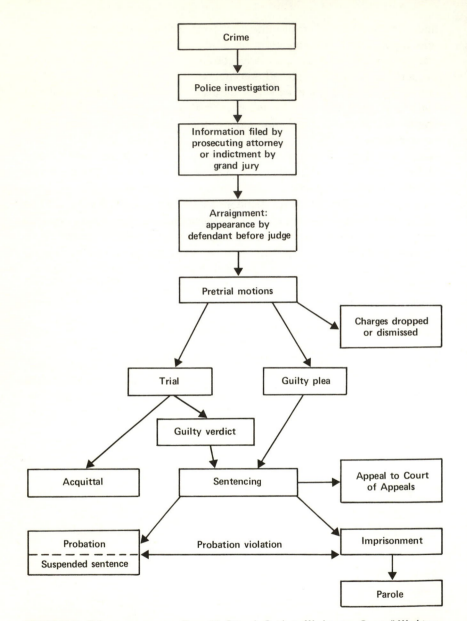

FIGURE 3. Felony case process. From "A Citizen's Guide to Washington Courts," Washington State Office of Administrator for the Courts.

person may plead guilty and consequently face sentencing. Once a judgment is made, the guilty person may be put on probation, may serve a jail term and/or pay a fine, or may go through the appellate process. If the charged person pleads not guilty, a trial date is set. At the end of the trial, a verdict is given of either guilty or not guilty. If the person is found not guilty, the charge is dismissed. If found guilty, the person faces probation and a jail term, and/or must pay a fine. This person, also, then may use the appellate process.

Felony case process is shown in Figure 3. When evidence exists that a crime may have been committed, the police begin their investigation. Then the information is either filed by the prosecuting attorney or given to the grand jury. If the evidence is sufficient for either the grand jury or the prosecuting attorney, the individual is arraigned or charged. Pretrial proceedings are generally informal in nature, and frequently cases are settled at this point.

If the person pleads guilty, sentencing of imprisonment, probation, and/or a fine is given. The appellate process is then made available. If the person pleads not guilty, the trial is set, the facts of the case are determined, the principles of law relating to those facts are applied, and a conclusion as to liability is reached.

If the verdict and judgment are guilty, the individual goes through the same sentencing process as in the guilty plea. If the verdict is not guilty, the person is acquitted.

TYPES OF COURTS

As indicated earlier, the type of court that hears a particular case depends upon the offense or complaint. In criminal cases, the type of court depends on the nature of the offense and where it occurs. In civil cases, it depends on the amount of money involved and where the parties reside. The jury and judge are neutral arbitrators of the evidence.

Courts are also classified as either lower or higher, inferior or superior. The lower or inferior courts refer to those of limited authority. The superior or higher courts have broader authority.[2]

There are three jurisdictions that belong only to *federal courts*. They are federal crimes, such as racketeering and bank robbery, constitutional issues, and civil action involving parties not living in the same state.

Figure 4 illustrates the Federal Court system. The United States Supreme Court is the highest court in the Federal Court system. Directly under the United States Supreme Court jurisdiction are the United States Court of Claims, the United States Court of Customs and Patent Office, and the United States Court of Appeals (or Circuit Courts). The last court directs the actions of the United States Federal District Courts and Tax Courts. It is important and impressive to remember that when a decision is made by the Supreme Court of the United States, it becomes the law for all citizens.

The pattern for *state courts* is similar to the pattern for federal courts. There are inferior or lower courts and a process of appeals.

Figure 5 illustrates the State Court system. The lower courts hear cases involving civil matters, small claims, housing, traffic, and some misdemean-

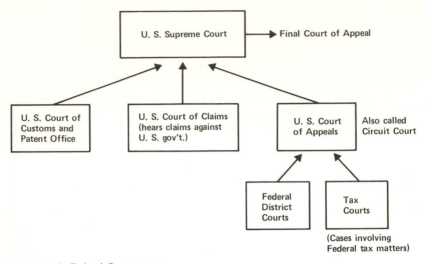

FIGURE 4. Federal Court system.

ors. The State Superior Court has general jurisdiction in all types of civil and criminal cases and, in some cases where the appeal is direct, the Court of Appeals is involved. The Court of Appeals may reverse, remand, modify, or affirm a decision of a lower court. The final route of appeal is to the State Supreme Court, the determination of which becomes the law of the state.

Each state, then, determines by statute the types of cases a particular court will hear and the maximum money value of the cases over which it has jurisdiction. In the event litigation does arise, physicians and their medical office employees most likely will find themselves in a state court regarding a civil matter. These civil matters may take place in probate and small claims courts.

In *probate court,* the physician may decide to initiate action on the collection of a bill owed by a deceased patient. The medical office employee represents the interests of the physician and attempts to locate the responsible person or party for the debt, whose name can be obtained from the deceased person's family, from the hospital, or from the mortuary. If you are unable to obtain a name from these sources, you should write or call the county seat in the county in which the estate is being settled. The county probate court recorder will provide information concerning the filing of the claim (in court, to the executor of the estate, or elsewhere), the proper forms to file, and when the claim must be submitted. It is best not to wait too long, as most states have a file period of from four to twelve months following the publication of notice in a newspaper by the administrator or executor.

Once the probate forms are ready to be mailed, send them by certified mail, return receipt requested. This establishes that the documents were received and by whom. The administrator will either accept or reject the

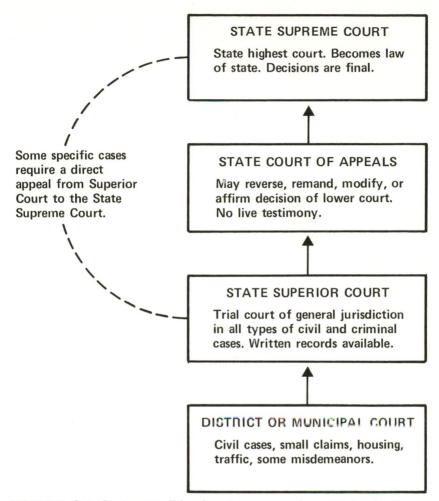

FIGURE 5. State Court system. Titles of courts vary across the country but this diagram generally applies.

claim. If it is accepted, payment will follow, but it may be delayed for months in the courts. If it is rejected, and the physician feels the bill is justified, a claim may be filed against the administrator within a designated amount of time, depending on the state. Be aware of your particular state's time limits.

Keep in mind that even though you may be hesitant to collect a deceased person's bill, the physician rendered services for the patient and deserves payment. Failure to file a claim may be construed by others as an admission of poor medical care on the part of the physician.

In the case of a delinquent account, the physician must initiate the action and may ask the bookkeeper or office assistant to take the delinquent account to *Small Claims Court,* where there is no representation by attorneys. In addition to the judgment of the amount owed, the plaintiff also may recover the costs of the suit. The wise office assistant will contact the clerk of Small Claims for instructions and information regarding the procedures to follow in Small Claims Court.

TRIAL PROCESS

A case may be tried before a judge or judge and jury. Usually trial courts have a jury, but the jury may be waived.

First, the jury, consisting of six to twelve people, must be selected. Usually the jury is randomly chosen from voter registration lists in the area. How they are further selected depends on the level of court, the type of case being tried, and upon local court rules. Once the jurors are selected, they are given the oath by a clerk or judge.

The trial procedure then begins. An opening statement is usually made by each attorney, first for the plaintiff, then for the defendant. Such statements outline the facts each party hopes to establish in the trial period. The plaintiff's attorney calls the first witness(es) and asks questions. This is considered *direct examination*. The defendant's attorney than *cross examines* the witness(es). This procedure continues until the plaintiff's entire case has been presented. The case for the defense is presented in the same manner. The direct and cross examinations reoccur. Then both attorneys *rest* their cases or indicate that no further evidence/testimony is to be given.

If it is a jury trial, the judge then instructs the jury on the law governing the case. The attorney for each party is allowed *closing arguments,* after which the judge charges the jury to reach a fair verdict based on the evidence presented. Then the jury is ushered from the courtroom to consider the case and reach a verdict. In a civil trial, five of six or ten of twelve jurors must agree. In a criminal trial, all twelve jurors must agree.

In civil court, the judge or jury finds for the plaintiff or for the defendant. If the verdict is found in favor of the defendant, the case is dismissed. If the plaintiff wins the case, a monetary settlement is usually allowed, the amount to be determined by the judge and jury.

In a criminal trial, if the defendant is found guilty, the judge imposes sentence. At sentencing, the court can commit the defendant to an institution or allow probation. At the end of trial, the judge informs the defendant of all rights to appeal. If the defendant is found not guilty, the case is dismissed.

SUMMARY

Again, this introduction to law does not pretend to provide all the necessary information the office employee may need. It is intended to provide basic information, not legal advice. It is important, however, for office employees to be knowledgeable in the law and to be aware of their professional responsibilities. Many activities in the medical office require legal knowledge, and this knowledge of the law may prevent illegal acts.

REFERENCES

1. HEMELT, MD AND MACKERT, ME: *Dynamics of Law in Nursing and Health Care*, ed 2. Reston, Boston, 1982, p 301.
2. IBID, p 305.

DISCUSSION QUESTIONS

1. As a medical receptionist, why is an understanding of the law important?

2. If you are involved in a civil case, describe the process the case will follow and identify factors determining the appropriate court.

3. Is a misdemeanor the same as a felony? Explain.

4. What influence did England have on the U.S. legal system?

5. List advantages and disadvantages of having a jury.

6. Currently, are there any cases under consideration in the United States Supreme Court that directly affect the medical office employee?

CHAPTER 2

BUSINESS MANAGEMENT FOR MEDICAL PRACTICE

LEARNING OBJECTIVES

Upon successful completion of this chapter, you will:

1. Define the four types of business management appropriate for medical practice.

2. List two advantages and two disadvantages of each of the four types of business management for both the physician and the employee.

3. Compare personnel needs in each of the four types of business management.

4. Define Health Maintenance Organization.

5. List two similarities and dissimilarities between the closed-panel HMO and the Individual Practice Association.

6. Identify the physicians' responsibilities to employees in business management.

DEFINITIONS

Group Practice. Type of business management in which three or more individuals organize to render professional service using the same equipment and personnel.

Health Maintenance Organization. Prepaid health care program rendered by participating physicians to an enrolled group of persons.

Partnership. Type of business management involving the association of two or more individuals who are co-owners of their business.

Professional Service Corporation. Specific type of corporation in which licensed individuals organize to render a professional service to the public. Such licensed individuals include physicians, lawyers, and dentists.

Sole Proprietorship. Type of business management owned by a single individual.

INTRODUCTION

Physicians may practice as sole proprietors, as partners in a partnership with other physicians, as shareholder-employees in a professional service corporation, or as members of a group practice. Which type of business management to enter is one of the first decisions made by physicians entering practice. Some physicians establish themselves in a sole proprietor business; others seek a partnership or form a service corporation when they first begin practice. Still others become members in a "group" organization for part or all of their professional careers. The business organization may change from time to time during physicians' careers, and will, in part, dictate a change in certain legal questions for them and their employees.

A change in business organization will impact office employees and their work. This will be seen in medical records, billing and accounting procedures, payroll, number and duties of employees, and benefits. Advantages and disadvantages of each type of organization are discussed. Office employees need to be aware of how the type of business organization affects them and their jobs.

SOLE PROPRIETOR

A "sole or single proprietorship" is a business owned by a single individual who receives all the profits and takes all the risks. It is the oldest form of business and is the easiest to start, operate, and dissolve. The physicians serving as sole or single proprietors of their medical offices will find advantages as well as disadvantages to this form of business management.

ADVANTAGES OF SOLE PROPRIETORSHIP

The advantages include simplicity of organization, being one's own "boss," being the sole receiver of all profits, and having few government regulations, low organizational costs, and great flexibility in operation.

To illustrate the advantages of the sole proprietorship, consider the example of a doctor who is able to establish practice in a community by purchasing or renting facilities, to make decisions without consideration of partners or other business colleagues, and to pay minimal organizational costs. The doctor also will not have to divide the profits with any other person and will be able to run the practice exactly as desired.

DISADVANTAGES OF SOLE PROPRIETORSHIP

There are disadvantages, however, to the single proprietorship. They include the fact that physicians may have difficulty raising sufficient capital to begin or expand the business. Medical equipment is among the most expensive of any type of equipment in a new business. It is possible that the profits of the business may be insufficient to allow for expansion. Also, physicians realize that if a business fails in a single proprietorship, their personal property may be attached and they may lose virtually all personal savings and possessions. Typically, the sole proprietor performs all, or at least most, of the managerial functions in the business. It is, therefore, common to find a sole proprietor working more than a standard 40-hour work week.[1]

Consider again this doctor, who has sufficient capital when entering practice to establish the office as a sole proprietorship. Initially, the system works well while the patient load is not high. However, the doctor soon finds time is a premium when working 70 to 80 hours a week carrying a full patient load while managing the business aspects of the practice as well.

CONSIDERATIONS FOR THE OFFICE ASSISTANT IN SOLE PROPRIETORSHIP

The sole proprietor will probably begin with just one assistant. This person will need training in all areas of administrative and clinical tasks to be performed in the office setting. While some assistants enjoy the opportunity to utilize all their skills in the "whole" operation, others may find it less attractive and prefer that the physician allow certain tasks to be sent out for completion. These tasks might include laboratory work, transcription, and correspondence. The sole proprietorship also may use the services of an accountant for quarterly and yearly tax reports.

The sole proprietorship offers little, if any, opportunity for advancement for its employees. Therefore, it is important that the physician reward employees with pay raises and benefits to encourage them to remain as employees. The physician must realize that it is usually an expense to hire a new employee and retrain that person for the task at hand. It is wise to select employees carefully on the basis of their education, training, and experience, to reward them sufficiently for their work, and to encourage them to stay a fair length of time with the practice. Many office assistants may prefer the sole proprietorship, however, because of the opportunity they have to make decisions and assume responsibility.

PARTNERSHIPS

Partnerships represent an association of two or more persons as co-owners of a business for profit. Most partnerships have only two or three members, but there is no limit to the number of individuals who may enter into a partnership. The organization may take many forms and is usually defined in a partnership agreement.

The partnership should have an agreement written and reviewed by an attorney. This agreement should include such items as the kind of business to be conducted or services to be performed, the kind of partnership being established, authority held by each partner, length of the partnership agreement, capital invested by each partner, description of how profits and losses are to be shared, how each partner is to be compensated, limitations on monetary withdrawals by a partner, accounting procedures to be followed, procedures for admitting new partners, dissolution of the partnership, and, of course, the signatures of the partners involved in the agreement.

ADVANTAGES OF PARTNERSHIPS

Some advantages of this form of business are easily recognized. Generally, there will be more financial strength than in the sole proprietorship. It is hoped that there will be additional managerial skill and a sharing of the workload. The organization of a partnership remains relatively simple, although somewhat more complicated than a sole proprietorship.

DISADVANTAGES OF PARTNERSHIPS

Disadvantages are that it takes more than one person to make the decisions. One cannot really be the "only" boss. If the partnership fails, usually each partner can be liable for the whole amount of the partnership debts, regardless of the size of the investment, unless otherwise specified in the partnership agreement. If one partner lacks personal finances to assume a full share of any loss, the other partners are required to make good the deficit.[2] Personality differences should be considered, as compatibility is important in any partnership. It may be advantageous to have a "trial period" that allows a partner to terminate or withdraw from the association or be asked to withdraw or terminate.

When a doctor is deciding how to establish practice, the partnership may be desirable. If it is an already established practice, it may require only a small capital investment in the beginning. This investment can be increased as the doctor becomes more financially secure. A sole proprietor often will turn to a partnership when the workload of the practice requires a second person to share the work. If the doctor does not wish to enter a partnership agreement, but needs additional help, another physician may be hired strictly on a salary basis. While this does not constitute a partnership, a contract may be desirable for the protection of each party.

CONSIDERATIONS FOR THE OFFICE ASSISTANT IN PARTNERSHIPS

A partnership should consider hiring more than one assistant in the office setting, because of the increased workload. Each partner may desire an assistant, but many tasks will be common to each and are best performed by one person. It is important for assistants to understand the partnership relationship and the line of authority. Open communication on the part of all members of the staff is essential. Otherwise, it is very easy to have each physician expecting an assistant to function as a member of the staff but not providing input as to how this should be done.

In addition, with more than one employee, both job advancement and job specialization are possible. For example, the newly formed partnership hiring a second assistant may want to name the first assistant office manager with a specific set of duties or to assign one to administrative tasks while the other performs clinical duties.

PROFESSIONAL SERVICE CORPORATIONS

A corporation is a legal entity that is granted many of the same rights enjoyed by individuals. These include the right to own, mortgage, and dispose of property, the right to manage its own affairs, and the right to sue and be sued.[3] Physicians in a professional corporation remain personally liable for their acts of medical malpractice.

Professional service associations or professional corporations are designed for professional persons such as physicians, lawyers, dentists, and accountants. These corporations can be identified by the letters S.C. (service corporation), P.C. (professional corporation), Inc. (incorporated), and P.A. (professional association), depending upon state law. The professional service corporation is the most intricate of all forms of medical practice.

ADVANTAGES OF PROFESSIONAL SERVICE CORPORATIONS

Advantages include the fact that contributions to pension and/or profit-sharing plans can be made for all employees including the physician. Such funds are deducted by the corporation from its taxable income, are invested, and accumulate in tax-free trusts until a future time of disbursement. Taxes are not paid on the funds until the time of their disbursement—usually at retirement, when the individual is in a lower tax bracket.

Another advantage is the corporate medical reimbursement plan. Medical and dental expenses of the employees can be paid by the professional corporation. These expenses are deductible to the corporation and nontaxable to the employee. This can result in substantial savings to both corporation and employee. Group term life insurance on a deductible premium basis is another advantage to be considered in a professional corporation. The professional corporation also may pay the malpractice premiums for physicians and other employees.[4]

DISADVANTAGES OF PROFESSIONAL SERVICE CORPORATIONS

When professional service corporations first became legal, many physicians eagerly incorporated only to discover there were some disadvantages. The complexity of the professional service corporation and its detailed requirements call for reliable, well-informed attorneys and accountants to advise the practice. This may make it more expensive than other forms of organization.

Physicians in professional service corporations have discovered that full participation in pensions, profit-sharing plans, and medical reimbursement plans is essential if full benefits of this form of organization are to be realized. It is important to have regular meetings and to reach agreement on organization, investments, pensions, and profit-sharing plans. This obviously complicates decision-making because more individuals are involved than in a sole proprietorship or most partnerships. It is often difficult for physicians to find the time to perform the functions required to run a corporation.

It should be noted that while a professional service corporation usually involves two or more physicians functioning in a group setting, it is possible for a sole proprietor to incorporate as a professional service corporation. The income of a single individual who incorporates needs to be sufficient to allow full participation in the benefits granted to the professional service corporation or such an arrangement is financially ineffectual.

CONSIDERATIONS FOR THE OFFICE ASSISTANT

The professional service corporation generally employs more assistants than a partnership or sole proprietorship. The possibility of being a part of a profit-sharing plan and having medical expenses covered by the corporation are attractive inducements to prospective employees. This form of practice usually provides ample opportunity for advancement and specialization. One person should be responsible for all personnel matters to enable a smooth-running organization.[5]

GROUP PRACTICE

There is still another option of medical practice available to today's physicians—joining a group. The American Medical Association defines group practice this way:

> Group medical practice is the application of medical services by three or more physicians formally organized to provide medical care, consultation, diagnosis, and/or treatment through the joint use of equipment and personnel, and with the income from medical practice distributed in accordance with methods previously determined by members of the group.[6]

There are three main types of group practice:

(1) *Single specialty,* providing services in only one field of practice or major specialty, for example, a group of pediatricians joining together in practice.
(2) *Multispecialty,* providing services in two or more fields of practice or major specialties, for example, a group of obstetricians/gynecologists and pediatricians joining together in practice.
(3) *Primary care group,* providing obstetricians/gynecologists, pediatricians, family practitioners, and internists.

Group medical practice generally operates on a fee-for-service basis, as does the practice of a physician in a sole proprietorship, a partnership, or a professional service corporation.

ADVANTAGES OF GROUP PRACTICE

Advantages to physicians in the group practices include a shared financial investment for diagnostic and therapeutic equipment, the opportunity of consultation with other physicians, little administrative responsibility for the practice (a group may actually employ a medical manager for the business side of the operation), and more family and recreation time because member-physicians in the group cover for one another. In addition, group practice may offer the intellectual and social stimulation desired by some physicians.

DISADVANTAGES OF GROUP PRACTICE

Disadvantages are also easily identified. Not every physician has the personality to function well in a group setting. A physician cannot act totally independently of the group and may feel a loss of freedom in such a situation. While the working hours may not be as long, the income also may not be as high as in solo practice. Working in a close relationship with colleagues on a daily basis may lead to personality clashes and differences of opinion.[7]

CONSIDERATIONS FOR THE OFFICE ASSISTANT

There will be more employees in a group situation than in the other forms of medical organization simply because of the larger staff of physicians. Physicians generally will have less responsibility for hiring and selecting personnel, which may be an advantage or a disadvantage, depending upon the physicians' personal preferences. An employee may choose employment in a group for many of the same reasons as those in the corporation. There may be less personalization in a larger group, depending upon the number of employees.

HEALTH MAINTENANCE ORGANIZATIONS

In recent years, another group form, the Health Maintenance Organization (HMO), has become increasingly well-known. Kaiser Foundation and Group Health Cooperative are examples of the HMO. Such groups contract with patients to provide comprehensive health care and preventive medicine for prepaid fees that entitle the subscriber to service during the duration of the contract. The HMO may be a closed-panel group with all its services under "one roof," or it may be an Individual Practice Association (IPA). The IPAs are less structured organizations and have been able to avoid the large start-up costs that face the closed-panel HMO.

The *closed-panel HMO* employs physicians who agree to work on a salary basis with other physicians and allied health personnel in providing total care to patients who contract with the HMO for its medical services. The *Individual Practice Association* allows physicians to maintain their private practices, charge their regular fees, and be reimbursed for the prepayment patients by a central IPA organization. Therefore, the physicians involved in an IPA organization may have many regular fee-for-service patients as well as patients who have prepaid for their services to an IPA organization that will, in turn, pay the physician. The IPA makes use of the primary-care-physician concept as a method of controlling costs. All medical care sought by a patient must be channeled through the primary care physician.

The advantage to physicians who practice in a closed-panel HMO is that the working hours will be regular, allowing for more personal time. Also, the HMO physician will not have to provide the building or equipment necessary for practice. This, of course, is not the case in the IPA, where the physician is still responsible for all equipment and building costs.

EMPLOYER'S RESPONSIBILITIES TO EMPLOYEES

In whatever style of operation physicians choose to practice, there are certain business responsibilities for employers. These include Federal, state, and local requirements for Social Security compensation protection and workers' compensation for all employees. Benefits will need to be considered. These could include any or all of the following: (1) uniform allowance, (2) paid parking, (3) medical benefits, (4) retirement benefits, (5) profit-sharing, (6) vacations and sick leave, (7) paid holidays and/or personal leave time, (8) professional improvement allowances, and (9) malpractice insurance.

As stated earlier in this chapter, it is important for physicians to realize the value of well-trained employees and to encourage employees to remain with the organization as long as possible.

Specific information about physicians' responsibilities to employees can be obtained from an accountant or attorney. County or state medical associations have information about requirements for setting up a practice and also have guidelines for employees. The American Medical Association has a booklet *Professional Corporations in Perspective,* OP-102, and a publication titled *Group Practice Guidelines,* OP-456, which can be ordered from AMA, Order Department, P.O. Box 821, Monroe, WI 53566.

SUMMARY

Physicians can open new practices, function as sole proprietors, be employed by other physicians on a straight salary basis, establish partnerships, become part of professional service corporations, or join any of the different types of group organizations. No one form of practice is better than another. All have advantages and disadvantages. The choice will depend on the individual personality and preference of the physicians. None should be entered into without advice and consideration from persons knowledgeable in the field who can offer valuable information for physicians to evaluate. The overriding factor for physicians to consider is what type of business organization will best permit them to serve their patients.

REFERENCES

1.   MAUSER, FF AND SCHWARTZ, JR, DJ: *American Business — An Introduction.* Harcourt, Brace & World, San Francisco, 1966, p 55.

2.   IBID, pp 56-58.

3.   IBID, p 62.

4.   ZIRKLE, TE: *Professional Corporations in Perspective.* American Medical Association, Monroe, WI, May 1978, pp 2-3.

5.   IBID, pp 10-11.

6.   AMERICAN MEDICAL ASSOCIATION: *The Business Side of Medical Practice.* Monroe, WI, 1979, p 9.

7.   IBID.

DISCUSSION QUESTIONS

1. What kind of business management exists in the office where you are employed or where you would be most interested in seeking employment?

2. Give reasons why physicians may choose a particular style of business management at different stages of their careers.

3. On a sheet of paper, make a column for the four kinds of business management. List as many advantages and disadvantages as you can for each. When you finish, determine if one kind is better than another.

4. Refer to question three. Add possible employee benefits available in each kind of business management. Select the kind most suitable to your needs and explain why.

5. You are offered a position in a HMO, but enjoy your present position of employment in a sole proprietorship. What must you consider in making a decision?

6. You are convinced that medical costs must be contained but are not certain that the closed-panel HMO is the answer. What are the alternatives?

CHAPTER 3

THE EMPLOYEES IN THE MEDICAL OFFICE

LEARNING OBJECTIVES

Upon successful completion of this chapter, you will:

1. List and define the four categories of medical office employees.

2. List and define the three categories of nurses found in a medical office. Compare their education and training.

3. Recall at least three examples of nonlicensed personnel in a medical office.

4. List two similarities and dissimilarities between:
   a. technician and technologist
   b. physician assistant and medical assistant.

5. Explain in a brief paragraph, professional liability in the employer-employee relationship.

DEFINITIONS

Certification. Documentation usually from a professional organization that an individual has met certain requirements set forth by that organization.

Laboratory Technician. Person who has graduated from a certificate program or associate degree program as a laboratory assistant. Either graduate works under the supervision of a physician or medical technologist in a laboratory.

Licensed Practical Nurse (LPN), also called **Licensed Vocational Nurse** (LVN). Person who has graduated from a one-year practical nurse vocational or college program and has passed the state licensing examination for practical or vocational nurses. An LPN or LVN works under the direct supervision of an RN or a physician.

Licensure. Legal permission, granted by state statutes, to perform specific acts; as a physician is licensed to practice medicine.

Medical Assistant (MA). Person who assists the physician in both administrative (front office) and clinical (back office) duties; education varies from on-the-job to two years in an accredited program for medical assisting.

Medical Technologist. Person who has graduated from a two- to four-year college or university program in medical technology that includes one year of clinical training in the laboratory.

Negligence. Doing some act that a reasonable and prudent physician would not do or the failure to do some act that a reasonable and prudent physician would do.

Nurse Practitioner (NP). Registered Nurse who has successfully completed additional training in a nurse-practitioner program. An NP can function alone or under the supervision of a physician in a medical facility.

Physician Assistant (PA). Person with one to four years of education in an approved program for PAs; a PA works under the license and supervision of the physician.

Reciprocity. An agreement by which two states recognize the licensing procedures of each other, consider them valid, and grant a license to practice.

Registered Nurse (RN). Person who has graduated from a one- to three-year nursing program, a two-year associate degree or three-year diploma, or a four- to five-year bachelor's degree program, and passed the state licensing examination for Registered Nurses. An RN works under the supervision of a physician.

Registration. An entry in an official record, listing names of persons satisfying certain requirements.

INTRODUCTION

The number and kinds of employees in the medical office will vary with the practice. Generally, the more specialized the practice, the more specialized the personnel. Employees in the medical office may fall into the following categories: (1) those who are licensed; (2) those who are registered; and

(3) those who are certified. There also may be employees who are none of the three.

Licensure is the strongest form of regulation. Licensed employees must obtain their licenses from the state authority prior to employment. A license establishes that the employee has met minimum standards required by law. Licensure of physicians will be discussed in the next chapter.

Registration is a process by which individuals in a particular health field are listed in a registry. This list is then available to health care providers. The state has little or no power over the registration process. There are two methods of registration. One occurs when individuals list their names in an official register of a health area in which they work. There is no power to deny employment to unlisted persons, however. The second requires a certain level of education and/or payment of a fee for registration. The only limiting factor here is that you cannot claim to be registered if you are not.[1]

Certification is probably the most common form of regulation and occurs when a particular organization warrants that the certified person has attained a certain level of knowledge and skill. Again, however, this does not prevent anyone without certification from practicing.

Licensed, certified, and registered persons may use appropriate symbols after their names to verify their credentials. Examples include the RN (Registered Nurse), CMA (Certified Medical Assistant), and MT (ASCP) Medical Technologist (American Society of Clinical Pathologists). Both certification and registration are voluntary. Licensure is mandatory.

Those who are not licensed, registered, or certified also are employed in medical offices. There is no professional organization regulating these employees. They may be trained on the job, or they may have professional training and education but have not attained certification or registration.

LICENSED PERSONNEL

A common employee in the medical office is the nurse. Training and education for nurses fall into three categories: Licensed Practical or Vocational Nurse, Registered Nurse, and Nurse Practitioner.

LICENSED PRACTICAL NURSE (LPN), ALSO CALLED LICENSED VOCATIONAL NURSE

Graduate Practical Nurses (GPNs) may take their state board examination to be licensed as a Licensed Practical Nurse or Licensed Vocational Nurse. GPNs have completed a one-year vocational education course at a community agency, a public vocational school, or a junior/community or senior college. The substance of this program includes elementary nursing practices and introductory educational courses. This nurse is considered a technician.

REGISTERED NURSE (RN)

Graduate nurses (GNs) from one of three educational preparations may take the state board examination to be licensed as a Registered Nurse:

1. *The Diploma Nurse*—generally a graduate of a hospital-based program of two or three years during which nurses engage in patient care and classroom work. Direct patient care and bedside experience are stressed.
2. *The Associate Degree Nurse*—a graduate of a junior/community college program that awards graduates an associate degree in nursing. The college provides the educational base and condenses the practical instruction into a two-year program.
3. *The Bachelor's Degree Nurse*—a graduate of a four- or five-year program that stresses the importance of general nursing education rather than hospital-based experience. Most administrative positions are held by bachelor's degree nurses as are the positions of public health and school nurse.

GNs sit for the same state board examination regardless of their educational preparation. The GPNs however, sit for a state board examination specifically commensurate with the work performed. The education and training received in all these programs emphasize hospital and/or nursing facility employment rather than office employment.

When the nurse passes the appropriate state examination, the LPN, LVN, or RN is conferred. This license is renewed each year by paying the required fee. Some states require continuing education units (CEUs) for license renewal. Continuing education includes seminars, workshops, college courses, independent studies, and approved on-the-job training. Nurses must keep a record of all successfully completed continuing education classes and submit proof of completion to the appropriate agency when renewing their licenses. All nurses should be knowledgeable of their state's requirements and recommendations. Employers of office nurses should have a procedure for checking licenses annually.

Nurses wishing to practice in another state must seek reciprocity in that state. Reciprocity occurs when one state recognizes the licensing procedure of another, considers it valid, and grants a license to practice. If there is no reciprocity process, the nurse must satisfy the state's licensure requirement.

NURSE PRACTITIONER (NP)

The Nurse Practitioner is a Registered Nurse (usually with a bachelor's degree) who has successfully completed additional training in a nurse practitioner program. Nurse practitioner education and training usually comprise four months to a year and may lead to a specific diploma or a master's degree. The graduate nurse practitioner then seeks national certification, which requires written and/or oral examination. The American Nurses Association grants the NP certification.

Nurse practitioners usually function independently in expanded nursing roles according to each state's nurse practice act. They may specialize and be certified in such specialties as pediatrics, geriatrics, midwifery, or emergency room. Nurse practitioners may examine, diagnose, and treat patients—acts formerly performed solely by physicians. This diagnosis and treatment often puts the nurse practitioner in the center of controversy with physicians.

The employment field for nurse practitioners is varied. For instance, they may be found in isolated areas of the country managing a clinic and providing total patient care. Or they may be found in public health in charge of family planning clinics. A nurse practitioner also may be found in a pediatrician's office responsible for the initial history, examination, and screening of patients who are then seen by the physician.

Physicians may choose to employ nurses because of their technical expertise in clinical areas. Few nurses, however, will have skills relating to the business aspect of the medical office or have the desire to function in that capacity.

NONLICENSED PERSONNEL

Generally, most office employees are nonlicensed. These individuals include Physician Assistants, Medical Assistants, Medical Technologists, and Medical Laboratory Technicians. Education and training varies widely among nonlicensed personnel. Many are certified and/or registered. All function under the supervision of the physician.

PHYSICIAN ASSISTANTS (PA)

Physician Assistants are usually totally under the control of the Medical Licensure board, and they practice under the supervision of the physicians who employ them. PAs themselves are not licensed. The educational requirements for the PA vary widely, from one to four years. Some programs require two years' undergraduate study in biology and behavioral science with some work experience in the health field prior to admittance to PA training. Two-year programs for PAs provide clinical and practical components covering anatomy and physiology, microbiology, pharmacology, and applied behavioral science courses. Four-year programs provide the student liberal arts and behavioral science courses. Classroom and supervised clinical instruction is common to both two- and four-year programs. Among tasks performed by PAs are interviewing patients, taking histories, doing routine physicals and laboratory tasks, treating burns, suturing and caring for cuts and wounds, changing dressings, making rounds in the hospital, and prescribing and administering medications—always under the supervision and control of their physician employers.

Nearly all states have enacted legislation affecting PAs. The laws either reconfirm the physician's authority over the PAs or vest authority in a state agency to establish rules for recognition of PAs. No state is known to license PAs, except Colorado, which licenses graduate Child Health Associates (a type of PA).

Graduates of accredited programs for PAs may apply to the National Commission on Certification for PAs for examination. The individual meeting the requirements is recognized as a PA-C, Physician Assistant Certified.[2]

Physicians may be restricted as to the number of PAs they may supervise. This is to insure that adequate supervision is available. PAs may be found in many areas. Most work with physicians in private solo or partnership practices, but PAs also work in a variety of hospital settings as well as in group practice situations.

MEDICAL ASSISTANTS

Medical Assistants are often confused with physician assistants. Both work under the supervision of physicians, but their duties are distinct. The medical assistant's versatility provides for efficient management of the entire office. While the medical assistant is a generalist, the role may be quite specific, depending upon the duties assigned.

Educational and training programs for the medical assistant are usually one or two years in a vocational or community or junior college awarding a certificate/diploma or associate degree. Programs include academic courses and clinical experience. Typically, the medical assistant receives training and education in both the front office (administrative) and the back office (clinical).

Medical assistants may apply for certification to the Certifying Board of the American Association of Medical Assistants. There are three examinations. The *Basic* examination covers all aspects of medical assisting. Two specialty examinations include *Administrative* and *Clinical*. Upon successful completion of the examinations, the appropriate initials may be used after the name. They are Certified Medical Assistant (CMA), Certified Medical Assistant-Administrative (CMA-A) and Certified Medical Assistant-Clinical (CMA-C).

The training and education of medical assistants specifically prepare them for employment in the medical office setting.

TECHNOLOGISTS

Technologists are nonlicensed personnel often found in medical offices and clinics. They differ from technicians in that technologists require little to no supervision and often supervise the technician. Examples include electroencephalographic, medical, nuclear medicine, radiation therapy, and surgical technologists. Of these technologists, the medical technologist is most likely to be found in the medical office and clinic.

Federal regulations to encourage quality control mandate that a medical technologist be in charge of medical laboratories. While medical laboratories are usually in hospitals, many physicians have private laboratories because immediate results from the laboratory tests play an important role in the detection, diagnosis, and treatment of many diseases.

Requirements for the medical technologist include a minimum of 90 semester hours or 135 quarter hours of academic credit from a college or university and 12 months' clinical training. The curriculum includes instruction in hematology, serology, clinical chemistry, and microbiology, emphasizing basic principles commonly used in diagnostic laboratory tests.

Upon graduation the medical technologist is encouraged to apply to the Board of Registry of the American Society of Clinical Pathologists to take the certification examination. Upon successful completion of this examination, medical technologists can use the initials MT (ASCP) following their names.[3] At least one state—California—requires licensure through a state board examination.

LABORATORY TECHNICIANS

Laboratory Technicians also are found in the medical office or clinic. Education is obtained through either a certificate program or an associate degree program.

The certificate program is 12 months, with classroom training. Upon graduation, application may be made to the Board of Registry of the American Society of Clinical Pathologists for the certification examination. Upon successful completion, the individual then becomes a *Certified Laboratory Assistant*, CLA(ASCP).

The associate degree program is two years of education and training in a junior or community college. The student applicant must meet certain prerequisites depending on the college. Academic courses are taught in conjunction with clinical experience. Upon graduation, application may be made to the Board of Registry of the American Society of Clinical Pathologists to sit for the certification examination. Upon successful completion of the examination, the individual becomes a *Medical Laboratory Technician*, MLT (ASCP).

The main difference between the two graduates is that the associate degree technician can discriminate between closely similar items and can correct the errors. This associate degree technician can perform complicated tests and can monitor quality-control programs.

Both MLTs and CLAs perform all routine procedures in hematology, serology, blood banking, urinalysis, microbiology, and clinical chemistry under the supervision of a qualified physician and/or medical technologist.[4]

OTHER EMPLOYEES

Other employees in the medical office setting not previously discussed include the medical receptionist, medical secretary, medical transcriptionist, bookkeeper, and insurance biller. The tasks performed by these individuals are no less important than the others mentioned, though they are not licensed, certified, or registered. Their training and education will vary from on-the-job to formal university education.

All employees of the medical office need to continue their education, no matter what their initial educational preparation. Obviously, continuing education will benefit not just the individual and employer but, more importantly, the welfare of patients.

State regulations vary and will continue to change as medicine becomes more specialized. In some states, medical assistants cannot perform venipuncture. Some states also regulate radiography and who can administer medications. It is important for physician-employers to understand regulations pertinent to those individuals in their employ. It is also the professional responsibility of the *employees* to understand regulations pertaining to their jobs. Practicing within the law is essential for the protection of patients, employers, and employees.

PROFESSIONAL LIABILITY

Professional liability exists for both employer and employee. Physicians are not only responsible for their own actions of negligence, but also are responsible for the negligent actions of their employees under the doctrine of *respondeat superior.* This is a Latin phrase that means "Let the master answer." Consider the case of a physician assistant who administers an allergy shot, dismisses the patient, and hastens on to the next task without keeping the patient under observation for 20 minutes. The patient collapses in the parking lot a few minutes later as a result of anaphylactic shock from the injection. The physician-employer is responsible for the negligence of the PA. The physician assistant also is liable and both can be sued.

The physician-employer also is responsible for assuring that all employees perform only those tasks within the scope of their knowledge and training. For example, when a physician instructs a medical assistant to draw blood from a patient in a state in which such an act is illegal, the physician is requesting an illegal act. In addition, the medical assistant who performs the illegal act is at fault. In some states, both the physician and the medical assistant could face criminal charges.

The physician's employee has a responsibility to question an order if there is good reason. If the order is not questioned, and negligence occurs as a result, both the physician and the employee are liable.

Professional liability is a concern of all allied health professionals, but is an even greater concern to physicians, who are in a position of higher authority. The next chapters look closely at those laws of special importance to physicians.

REFERENCES

1. ANNAS, GJ, GLANTZ, LH, AND KATZ, F: *The Rights of Doctors, Nurses, and Allied Health Professionals.* Avon Books, New York, 1981, p 44.
2. AMERICAN MEDICAL ASSOCIATION: *Allied Health Educational Directory,* ed 10. Monroe, WI, 1981, p 70.
3. IBID, p 78.
4. IBID, p 76.

DISCUSSION QUESTIONS

1. Case A: Solo Family Practitioner is setting up a practice in a small, rural community.

   Case B: Six physicians are entering a group practice in a city of 40,000. Specialties include OB/GYN, Family Practice, Internal Medicine, and Pediatrics.

   What number and kinds of employees would you recommend in Case A? In Case B? Explain your choices.

   Discuss the professional liability of the solo practitioner and your selected employees. Discuss the professional liability of the six physicians in group practice and your selected employees.

2. What kind of medical practice is most likely to utilize a:
   a) physician assistant
   b) medical assistant?

3. Discuss the differences among licensure, certification, and registration.

CHAPTER 4

THE IMPORTANCE OF THE LAW TO THE PHYSICIAN

LEARNING OBJECTIVES

Upon successful completion of this chapter, you will:

1. Identify four common requirements for a physician to be licensed.

2. Identify three conditions in which a physician's license may be revoked.

3. List the three steps necessary for obtaining a narcotics registration.

4. Describe in outline form the office procedures to follow for administering and dispensing of controlled substances.

5. List the five schedules of controlled substances and give an example of each.

6. Define general and professional liability for physicians.

7. Define negligence and malpractice.

8. Restate in your own words the importance of professional liability insurance.

9. Outline the arbitration process for settling a malpractice suit.

10. Recall six methods of malpractice prevention.

11. Define Good Samaritan laws.

DEFINITIONS

Administer a Drug. To instill a drug into the body of a patient.

Arbitration. Settlement of dispute by neutral person hearing both sides before making a decision.

Bond. A legal obligation to pay specific sums.

Burglary. Breaking and entering with intent to commit a felony.

Controlled Substances Act. Federal law regulating the administration, dispensing, and prescription of particular substances that are categorized in five schedules.

Dispense a Drug. To deliver controlled substances in a bottle, box, or some other container to the patient. Under the Controlled Substances Act, the definition also includes the administering of controlled substances.

"Going Bare." Slang term for having no malpractice insurance coverage.

Medical Malpractice. Professional negligence of physicians.

Negligence. Doing some act that a reasonable and prudent physician would not do or the failure to do some act that a reasonable and prudent physician would do.

Prescribe a Drug. To issue a drug order for a patient.

Theft. Actual taking and carrying of someone else's personal property without consent or authority.

Tickler File. A periodic reminder to do specific tasks on schedule; usually daily, weekly, or monthly.

INTRODUCTION

Without an understanding of laws that directly relate to physicians, the medical office employee may inadvertently cause difficulties. Therefore, it is important to consider those laws and regulations that directly influence the actions of medical office employees and physicians.

The law is, at times, both complicated and vague. It is not possible to cover in this book all parts of the law as it may affect physicians and employees. Only laws related to the practice of medicine in an office or clinic are emphasized.

MEDICAL PRACTICE ACTS

Medical Practice Acts are state statutes that define the practice of medicine, describe methods of licensure, and set guidelines for suspension or revocation of a license. All 50 states have such statutes to protect their citizens from harm by unqualified persons practicing medicine.

LICENSURE

Physicians must be licensed in the United States in order to practice medicine. States differ in their licensing requirements. The more common requirements include graduation from an accredited medical school, completed internship, good moral character, and successful completion of the Federation Licensing Examination (FLEX).[1] Foreign-trained and -educated physicians are required to pass the FLEX examination or an equivalent test.

Physicians who choose to practice in more than one state must satisfy the license requirements of each state. This may be done by requiring physicians to pass each state's exam, reviewing their past practices, or through reciprocity. Reciprocity may be granted when one state recognizes the licensing procedure of another, considers it valid, and issues a license to practice.

Not all physicians need to be licensed by the state where they are employed. These include physicians practicing medicine in the Armed Forces, in Veterans Administration facilities, and with the U.S. Public Health Service. Physicians engaged strictly in research and not practicing medicine need not have a license.

LICENSE RENEWAL

Physicians renew their licenses periodically, usually upon payment of a fee. Notice will be received by the physician at the time of renewal. Documentation of continuing education units (CEUs) is increasingly becoming a requirement for renewal. Specific state requirements differ, but 50 hours a year is standard.[2] Appropriate credits will be identified in the statutes and may include (1) reading of books, papers, publications, (2) teaching health professionals, (3) attending approved courses, workshops, and seminars, and (4) self-instruction.[3]

Physicians' employees may be responsible for record-keeping of the continuing education activities. It is wise to have your state's requirements on file and to be able to verify the credits as required.

LICENSE REVOCATION AND SUSPENSION

Three conditions that may dictate that the license to practice be revoked or suspended are (1) conviction of a crime, (2) unprofessional conduct, and (3) personal or professional incapacity.[4]

Conviction of a crime is a more obvious reason for license revocation than is unprofessional conduct or personal or professional incapacity. Examples of *unprofessional conduct* may include the falsification of any records regarding licensing, dishonesty, impersonating another physician, and treating a disease with any "secret remedy." *Personal or professional incapacity* includes chronic alcoholism, drug abuse, continuing to practice when severe physical limitations prevent adequate care, and practicing outside the scope of training.

Usually charges against physicians are made by the physician's licensing board. In all states the basic procedure for disciplinary action is nearly identical. Most boards are required to give the physician licensee sufficient notice of the charges, allowing the licensee legal counsel and a hearing. The board then investigates, prosecutes, makes a judgment, and sentences. Some states have empowered their licensing board to suspend a license to practice, on a temporary basis, without a hearing when the physician poses an immediate threat.

BUSINESS LICENSE

Some communities require a business or occupational license before allowing an office to be opened for the practice of medicine. Physicians should check with county and city clerks to see if a license is required and what procedures are to be followed. An annual renewal fee may be necessary.

NARCOTICS LAWS AND REGULATIONS

The Drug Enforcement Administration (DEA) of the Department of Justice is responsible for enforcement of the Comprehensive Drug Abuse Prevention and Control Act of 1970, Title II—more commonly known as the Controlled Substances Act.[5] These drugs are controlled because of their potential for abuse and dependence. Drug abuse is discussed in Chapter 5. The Controlled Substances Act lists controlled drugs in five schedules (I, II, III, IV, V), which are discussed in detail later in this section.

The Controlled Substances Act and United States Code of Federal Regulations are important to all physicians, but are especially pertinent to those who will be administering, prescribing, or dispensing to patients drugs that are listed in the five schedules. Requirements for physicians include registration, record-keeping, inventory, and proper security.

Registration is with the DEA, Registration Section, P.O. Box 28083, Central Station, Washington, D.C. 20005. Initial application is made on DEA Form 224, which can be obtained from the above address or any DEA Regional Office (see Figure 6). A number is assigned to each legitimate handler, and registration is renewed annually. Generally, a registration application, DEA Form 226, will be mailed by DEA to the registered physician approximately 60 days before the expiration date of the registration each year. If the application is not received within 45 days before the

North Eastern Regional Office
555 West 57th Street
New York, NY 10019
(212) 399—5151
   Canada, Montreal & Toronto
   Connecticut
   Delaware
   Maine
   Massachusetts
   New Hampshire
   New Jersey
   New York
   Pennsylvania
   Rhode Island
   Vermont

South Eastern Regional Office
8400 N.W. 53rd Street
Miami, FL 33166
(305) 591—4870
   Alabama
   Arkansas
   Florida
   Georgia
   Kingston, Jamaica
   Louisiana
   Maryland
   Mississippi
   North Carolina
   Puerto Rico
   South Carolina
   Tennessee
   Virginia
   Washington, D.C.

South Central Regional Office
1880 Regal Row
Dallas, TX 75235
(214) 767—7203
   Arizona
   Colorado
   New Mexico
   Oklahoma
   Texas
   Utah
   Wyoming

North Central Regional Office
1800 Dirksen Federal Building
219 South Dearborn Street
Chicago, IL 60604
(312) 353—7875
   Illinois
   Indiana
   Iowa
   Kansas
   Kentucky
   Michigan
   Minnesota
   Missouri
   Nebraska
   North Dakota
   Ohio
   South Dakota
   West Virginia
   Wisconsin

Western Regional Office
Suite 900
350 South Figueroa Street
Los Angeles, CA 90017
(213) 688—2650
   Alaska
   California
   Canada, Vancouver
   Guam
   Hawaii
   Idaho
   Montana
   Nevada
   Oregon
   Washington

FIGURE 6. DEA domestic regional offices.

registration expiration, notice of such fact and a request for forms must be made in writing to the Registration Section of the DEA.[6]

A separate DEA registration is granted for each of several business activities and is different for residents, interns, and foreign physicians. Therefore, physicians should check with the DEA to make certain the proper registration is made. The initial registration fee is $5 as is the annual registration fee. Two helpful booklets are the *United States Code of Federal Regulations, Title 21,* Parts 1300 to End, Office of the Federal Register, National Archives and Records Service, General Services Administration, Revised April 1, 1981 (available at Federal government bookstores), and *Physician's Manual,* DEA, Office of Public Affairs, April 1978 (available at your regional DEA office).

Record-keeping is required by physicians for the *dispensing* of narcotic and non-narcotic drugs to patients. The records must be kept for two years and are subject to DEA inspection. The record must include the following information:

1. Full name and address of each patient to whom drug was given.
2. Date drug was given.
3. Name and quantity of drug given.
4. Method of dispensing.
5. Reason for drug (may be in patient's chart).[7]

Physicians who only *prescribe* narcotic and/or non-narcotic drugs are not required to keep the detailed record stated above.

Inventory is required of physicians who regularly engage in dispensing drugs. Inventory must be taken upon the date of registration and every two years thereafter. The following is required:

1. Name, address, and DEA registration number.
2. Date and time of inventory, e.g., opening or closing of business.
3. Signature of person(s) taking inventory.
4. Inventory record to be on file for at least two years.
5. Separate record required for Schedule II drugs.[8]

Security is necessary for controlled substances. These drugs must be kept in a locked cabinet or safe that is substantially constructed. Any loss is to be reported to the Regional DEA office and local law enforcement.[9]

DRUG SCHEDULES

All controlled substances are divided into five schedules. A complete list should be obtained from the Regional Office of the DEA or can be found in the *Code of Federal Regulations, Title 21.* A brief summary follows.

Schedule I: This schedule lists drugs of high potential for abuse and that have no current accepted medical use. Schedule I drugs will be used by physicians only for purposes of research, approved by the Food and Drug Administration and the DEA, and only after a separate DEA registration as a researcher is obtained.[10] The manufacture, importation and sale of these drugs is prohibited. However, some states have enacted legislation to permit the use and possession of marijuana for certain medical patients.

Examples: heroin, marijuana, and LSD.

Schedule II: These drugs have current accepted medical use in the United States, but with severe restrictions. There is with these drugs a high potential of abuse that may lead to severe psychological or physical dependence.

Examples: *Narcotics:* morphine, codeine, Percodan.

Non-narcotics: amphetamines, Ritalin, Nembutal, and Quaalude.

When Schedule I and II drugs are ordered, the physician must use a special order form (DEA Form 222) that is preprinted with the physician's name and address. The form is issued in triplicate. One copy is kept in the physician's file while the remaining copies are forwarded to the supplier who, after filling the order, keeps a copy and forwards the third copy to the nearest DEA office.[11]

Prescription orders for Schedule II drugs must be written and signed by the physician. Some states, by law, require special prescription blanks with more than one copy. The physician's registration number must appear on the blank. The order may not be telephoned in to the pharmacy except in an emergency, as defined by the DEA. A prescription for Schedule II drugs may not be refilled.[12]

Schedule III. These drugs have less potential for abuse than substances in Schedule I and II. They have accepted medical use for treatment in the United States, but abuse may lead to moderate or low physical dependence or high psychological dependence.

Examples: *Narcotics:* various drug combinations containing codeine and paregoric.

Non-narcotics: amphetamine-like compounds and butabarbital.

Schedule IV: These drugs have a lower potential for abuse than those in Schedule III and have accepted medical use in the United States, but their abuse still may lead to limited physical or psychological dependence.

Examples: Chloral hydrate, meprobamate, Librium, Valium, and Darvon.

Schedule III and IV drugs require either a written or oral prescription by the prescribing physician. If authorized by the physician on the initial prescription, the patient may have the prescription refilled up to the number of refills authorized, which may not exceed five times or beyond six months from the date that the prescription was issued.[13]

Schedule V: These drugs have less potential for abuse than drugs in Schedule IV, and their abuse may be limited to physical or psychological dependence. Refills are the same as for drugs in Schedules III and IV.

Examples: This schedule includes cough medications containing codeine and antidiarrheals such as Lomotil.

According to the law, the only person authorized to issue prescriptions is the registrant. A prescription issued by the physician may be communicated to the pharmacist by the medical office employees. This regulation may be less restrictive for medications *not* in the Controlled Substances Act.

If your state requires triplicate prescription blanks, they will be used for prescribing drugs. These are not to be confused with the Form DEA 222 described earlier for the ordering of Schedule I and II drugs. The triplicate blanks will be furnished by the state, and the regulations should be followed.

All prescriptions for controlled substances must be dated and signed on the day issued, bearing full name and address of the patient and the name, address, and DEA registration number of the physician. The prescription must be written in ink or typewritten and must be signed by hand by the physician.[14]

Physicians must know the laws of their state on controlled substances. The state regulations may be more strict than Federal regulations and may require a separate state registration.

Narcotics laws should be studied carefully by any physician who opens an office. *The Code of Federal Regulations, Title 21,* mentioned earlier, should be obtained from the nearest Federal government bookstore and studied carefully before handling of controlled substances in the medical office. A listing of the DEA regional offices appears in Figure 6.

GENERAL LIABILITY

Physicians engaged in business must be aware of their liability—general as well as professional. General liability includes liability for auto, theft, fire, and employees' safety. Professional liability concerns physicians' professional relationships with patients.

Office employees may be involved in payments of insurance premiums and submission of claims or in the establishment of physicians in practice. An understanding of physicians' general liability will be a helpful asset to any employer.

BUILDING

Physicians are responsible for the building and grounds where their business is conducted. If a person should be injured on those premises, physicians may be held legally responsible. It is wise, therefore, for physicians to carry liability insurance on the premises.

AUTO

Aside from personal auto insurance, physicians may want to consider non-owner liability insurance. Such a plan protects the physician-employers if an employee has an automobile accident while performing some duty related to the business. For physicians who commonly ask their employees to make a bank deposit on their way home or to deliver the monthly statements to the post office, such protection is wise when an auto is used. It makes no difference whose car an employee drives.[15]

THEFT / FIRE / BURGLARY

It is important to have protection against theft, fire, or burglary on the building as well as on equipment and furniture. Two types of fire insurance are most common. A co-insurance plan dictates that the owner is responsible for payment of a certain percentage of the loss—20 percent, 30 percent, and so forth. A second plan covers not only the loss but the replacement costs. The latter is, of course, more expensive, but more beneficial in the case of loss.[16]

Cost of protection from burglary and theft will depend upon location and the amount of money or valuables kept on the premises. It is wise to have little money on hand even though most burglary attempts are made for the purpose of taking narcotics. A discussion with insurance agents will identify proper protection.

Some physicians also may insure their accounts receivable, which would be nearly impossible to recover in case of fire or loss. It is best to place these items in a fireproof cabinet or safe at the end of each working day to prevent their loss even if insured.

EMPLOYEES' SAFETY

Physicians are expected to provide a safe place of employment for their employees. Safety requirements vary from state to state. Some of the variables include 1) the number of employees, 2) the type of employment, and 3) the safety record of the business. It is wise to check with the state agency administering such safety regulations, Workers' Compensation, and state medical association to determine responsibility in this area.

BONDING

Physicians may wish to "bond" employees who are handling financial records and money in the medical office. The purchase of a bond for a certain amount in an employee's name insures that physicians will recover the amount of the loss, up to the amount of the bond, in case the employee embezzles funds. This may be especially important when physicians do not have the time to spot-check financial transactions made by employees. It is a good idea during the interview of a prospective employee to determine if the candidate is "bondable."

PROFESSIONAL LIABILITY

Professional liability includes all possible civil and criminal liability that physicians can incur as a result of performing their professional duties. Criminal liability is discussed in Chapter 6. The focus here is civil liability. Failure to perform professional duties competently is *negligence*. More specifically, *negligence* is performing an act that a reasonable and prudent physician would not perform *or* the failure to perform an act that a reasonable and prudent physician would perform. *Gross negligence* generally refers to a high degree of negligence. *Contributory negligence* implies that more than one person may have contributed to the negligence. Negligence, as defined above, and *malpractice* are the same. Further details of the physician's liability, including negligence, are discussed in the next chapter.

Professional negligence is more easily prevented than defended. It should be obvious that physicians do not wish to be found negligent or become involved in a malpractice suit of any kind. However, patients are more aware today of their rights than ever before. In some cases, patients have been awarded as much as one million dollars in suits against physicians. It is imperative, therefore, for physicians to protect the physician-patient relationship at all times and to be above reproach in the performance of all duties.

In the event of a malpractice suit, physicians will find it an advantage to be protected by professional liability insurance.

PROFESSIONAL LIABILITY INSURANCE

The need for physicians to carry professional liability insurance is obvious for numerous reasons. The most important, perhaps, is financial protection. A physician "going bare," without insurance, would have to pay any court costs, damages, and attorney fees personally if a malpractice suit is lost.

Physicians need liability insurance protection whether they are employees or employers. For example, employment in a corporation, an HMO, or a hospital does not guarantee professional liability coverage. Many employers or institutions carry professional liability insurance merely on themselves or the institution, not on their employees. In some cases, patients sue both the employer *and* the employee. The employer's insurance company could, in turn, sue the employee. If employees are covered by an employer's liability policy, they should be specifically named. Employees may choose to carry their own professional liability coverage. For example, medical assistants who are members of the American Association of Medical Assistants (AAMA) may purchase professional and personal liability insurance through the organization.

As an employer, physicians need professional liability insurance, mainly because of the doctrine of *respondeat superior* (see Chapter 3). Here the physician may not be directly negligent, but liable because of the acts of employees.

Another reason for carrying professional liability insurance is because the physician may be asked for medical advice or assistance from friends or neighbors in a "casual situation." For example, at an outdoor barbecue, a neighbor may ask the physician, "I have this pain in my lower back. What should I do?" Or in the case of strangers, medical care may be emergent,[17] and the physician is the only one available. An employer's or institution's policy probably will not cover the physician in these situations. Good Samaritan Laws as they relate to professional liability will be discussed later.

The kind and amount of liability coverage a physician has will vary according to the type of practice, the community economic level, whether the specialty is considered a high risk, and if the patients are claims-conscious.[18] Most professional liability policies, however, should address the following: (1) What the insurer will pay, (2) effective policy dates, (3) the power of the insurer in obtaining legal counsel, (4) the power of the insurer in seeking settlement, (5) what costs are covered, and (6) how payment is to be made. The policy will specify monetary limits for each claim. For example, a policy may have professional medical liability of $1,000,000 for each claim and $3,000,000 aggregate as a total amount.

The cost of liability insurance is extremely high, ranging anywhere from $10,000 to $75,000 per year for a physician. In the 1970s when malpractice litigation was at its peak, many major insurance companies stopped offering the coverage. Many of those remaining companies increased their premiums to survive.[19]

Physicians found it difficult to pay the high premiums and sought other professional liability insurance or, in some states, physicians banded together to form their own companies to offer lower premiums. Medical societies have formed their own insurance companies. There are also major insurance carriers working with state medical societies to offer adequate coverage at lower premiums.

Another plan has been for physicians to purchase professional liability insurance for an amount less than advised or to change their practice to be within the coverage of insurance that can be afforded.

Some physicians and institutions have tried solving the malpractice dilemma by the initiation of arbitration. Here the patient voluntarily agrees, in advance, with the physician and/or institution to permit a neutral person or persons to arbitrate the case. Usually both the patient and the doctor select the arbitrators. In some instances, the arbitrators are preselected. The arbitrators then make a decision, based on established rules and statutes. Once a decision is made, the only action the courts can take is to determine whether the decision was fair. Arbitration usually saves time and money, and it may be more fair as well as more private.[20]

MALPRACTICE PREVENTION

Generally, if a healthy patient-physician relationship exists, malpractice suits are not likely to occur. Some helpful guidelines to prevent malpractice further include:

1. Perform no illegal acts, nor allow employees to do so.
2. Comply with state regulations and statutes.
3. Keep the office safe and the equipment in readiness.
4. Practice asepsis.
5. Log telephone calls. Return all calls to patients within a reasonable time.
6. Avoid treating patients via phone.
7. Put verbal instructions in writing and give a copy to the patient.
8. Do not criticize other practitioners.
9. Be sure all diagnostic test results are seen and initialed by the physician before filing.
10. Do not keep patients waiting for appointments for more than 20 minutes.
11. Select employees carefully and encourage the "team approach."
12. Keep all matters relating to patient care confidential.
13. Discuss patients' fees prior to treatment.
14. Have employees follow up on missed or canceled appointments.
15. Treat patients equally.
16. Never guarantee a cure.
17. Continue to grow professionally.
18. Secure informed consent as much as possible.
19. Listen to patients.
20. Formally document (a) withdrawing from a case, and (b) discharging a patient.
21. Carefully follow the Controlled Substances Act. Document all information required.
22. Keep accurate records.
23. Limit practice to scope of training, and to a manageable number of patients.

GOOD SAMARITAN LAWS

Good Samaritan statutes exist in all fifty states, yet their content varies widely with regard to who is protected, the standard of care required, and the circumstances under which protection is provided. The statute itself is a legal doctrine meant to encourage physicians and health care professionals to render emergency first aid treatment to accident victims without liability for negligence. It does not apply to an emergency arising in a clinic, hospital, or office where the patient-physician relationship exists.

The statutes mainly speak to physicians, but many also address other health care professionals. A few statutes will include laypersons. It must be kept in mind that in most states, no one, including physicians and health care professionals, has the legal obligation to stop and/or render first aid in a life-threatening situation. Most Good Samaritan statutes merely attempt to protect the physician or health care professional who does stop and acts "in good faith" and "without gross negligence." In Vermont, you *must* be a Good Samaritan or face a penalty,[21] whereas in Massachusetts, legislation states that physicians must administer emergency treatment to the best of their ability.[22]

The majority of Good Samaritan statutes are poorly written and leave many unanswered questions. Not many define the following: What is an emergency? What is care rendered gratuitously? Where and to what extent can care be given to be covered by the statute?

Many health care professionals are reluctant to render aid in an emergency. Reasons for this attitude may be the poorly written laws, legal and professional advice that says, "Beware," and the fear that the situation may require skills outside of their training and education. Perhaps, also, the health care professional is as anxious not to "get involved" as is the layperson. The risk of liability, however, has been grossly exaggerated. No successful lawsuits have ever been filed against a Good Samaritan physician or nurse.[23]

It is advisable for all health care professionals and their employees to know their Good Samaritan laws and specifically what and whom they address. The ethical issue also must be considered. The American Medical Association in the Principles of Medical Ethics states that physicians should respond to any requests for assistance in an emergency. Certainly the legal and ethical ramifications of rendering aid in an emergency should be considered before an emergency presents itself. While the health care professional may feel inadequate and unprotected in an emergency, the general public considers such a professional to be far more qualified than any layperson appearing on the scene.

Health care professionals who do render aid in an emergency should remember to treat within the scope of their training and to give adequate care in light of the circumstances. They should also take comfort in the fact that the chance of a lawsuit is slim.

CONSIDERATIONS FOR MEDICAL OFFICE EMPLOYEES

Employees will want to maintain a tickler file of all important dates to recall. These include due dates for license renewals, insurance premiums, and narcotics registrations. Established patterns must be maintained for drug inventory and record-keeping. Detailed descriptions and examples of such activities in the office's procedural manual are most helpful.

Employees are generally the first contact patients have with their physicians. Courtesy, and a genuine "I care" attitude will strengthen the physician-patient relationship. Employees can be of real assistance to physicians by reminding them of phone messages to return and by seeing that all pertinent matters are tended to by the end of the day.

Physicians should be told of patients who are angry or upset with any office functions. Most patients feel that a wait of more than 20 minutes for the doctor is unnecessary. Therefore, any delay should be explained honestly.

Physicians and their employees must function as teams in keeping one another informed of the needs of the patients they both serve.

REFERENCES

1. ANNAS, GJ, GLANTZ, LH, AND KATZ, BF: *The Rights of Doctors, Nurses, and Allied Health Professionals.* Avon Books, New York, 1981, p 6.

2. FREDERICK, PM AND KINN, ME: *The Medical Office Assistant.* WB Saunders, Philadelphia, 1981, p 52.

3. DIVISION OF PROFESSIONAL LICENSING: *The Law Relating to the Practice of Medicine.* Department of Licensing, Olympia, WA, January, 1979, p 23.

4. FREDERICK, p 52.

5. DRUG ENFORCEMENT ADMINISTRATION: *Drugs of Abuse.* US Government Printing Office, Washington DC, 6:2, 1980, p 2.

6. DRUG ENFORCEMENT ADMINISTRATION: *Physician's Manual.* US Department of Justice, Washington DC, April 1978, p 6.

7. FREDERICK, p 405.

8. DRUG ENFORCEMENT ADMINISTRATION: *Controlled Substances Inventory List.* US Department of Justice, Washington DC, 1979, p 2.

9. *Physician's Manual,* pp. 16–17.

10. OFFICE OF THE FEDERAL REGISTER: *Code of Federal Regulations, No. 21, Parts 1300 to End.* Washington DC, April 1981, p 6.

11. IBID, p 66.

12. *Drugs of Abuse,* pp 3–4.

13. IBID.

14. *Physician's Manual,* p 13.

15. AMERICAN MEDICAL ASSOCIATION: *The Business Side of Medical Practice*. Monroe, WI, 1979, p 25.

16. IBID.

17. CREIGHTON, H: *Law Every Nurse Should Know,* ed 3. WB Saunders, Philadelphia, 1975, p 253.

18. *The Business Side of Medical Practice,* p 24.

19. IBID.

20. FREDERICK, p 55.

21. CREIGHTON, p 104.

22. ANNAS, p 105.

23. IBID.

DISCUSSION QUESTIONS

1. A physician is coming into your established practice from another state. What must be done about licensure and narcotics registration?

2. Clarence calls requesting a refill for Percodan. Your records show that he has not been seen by the physician for almost a year. The doctor is away from the office for a week. What will you do? Consider the legal implications.

3. You've become the medical assistant for an orthopedic surgeon opening a new practice. Describe the types of liability insurance that will be needed and determine appropriate amounts.

4. Why would a physician in a medical office or clinic have the bookkeeper bonded?

5. When interviewing for a job in a medical office that bears much responsibility, you learn that the office professional liability insurance does not cover employees. What options are open to you?

6. Under what circumstances might a physician decide not to render emergency aid?

CHAPTER 5

PUBLIC DUTIES

LEARNING OBJECTIVES

Upon successful completion of this chapter, you will:

1. List seven areas of public duties for physicians.

2. Discuss, in your own words, the importance of filling out birth and death certificates.

3. Identify three circumstances in which a county coroner or medical examiner would be called to investigate a death.

4. Recall four items necessary in reporting:
   a. communicable diseases
   b. suspected child abuse.

5. Identify four professions the practitioners of which are required to report suspected child abuse.

6. Explain, in your own words, the drug abuse problem.

7. List four possible solutions for preventing drug abuse in the medical office.

DEFINITIONS

Autopsy. Examination by specially trained medical personnel of the body after death to determine cause of death or pathological conditions.

Coroner. An official, usually elected, who investigates death from sudden, unknown, or violent causes; may or may not be a physician.

Drugs.

    a. *Darvon:* mild to moderate pain reliever, has potential for abuse and dependency.

    b. *Librium:* tranquilizer for relief of wide range of emotional disorders including anxiety, tension, and withdrawal symptoms of acute alcoholism.

    c. *Meprobamate:* tranquilizer for relief of anxiety and tension. Promotes sleep in tense, anxious patients. Also marketed as: *Equanil, Meprospan,* and *Miltown.*

    d. *Valium:* prescribed for a wide variety of problems to provide relief from tension, anxiety, and skeletal muscle spasms.

Notifiable/Reportable Disease. A disease that concerns the public welfare and requires reporting to the proper authority. A potentially pathological condition that may be transmitted directly or indirectly from one individual to another.

Notifiable/Reportable Injury. An injury that concerns the public welfare and requires reporting to the proper authority; for example, injuries resulting from gun or knife wounds.

INTRODUCTION

Some details of many duties of physicians will become the responsibility of the medical office employees. Physicians, as licensed professionals, have statutory and regulatory requirements they must follow. Reports of births, stillbirths, deaths, communicable diseases, specific injuries, child and drug abuse are a few such examples. Report requirements vary among states. To become familiar with your particular state's reporting requirements, refer to the state's statutes and administrative regulations, which are available in most county libraries. In addition, it is a good idea for medical office employees to contact the local and state medical societies, the health department, and local law enforcement for reporting forms and information.

Gathering and reporting statistical data and information may become an impersonal task, but physicians and their staff need to remember that these data represent individuals. Therefore, the task is a personal matter. Deaths, rapes, and abuse are sensitive issues. Individuals involved need special care.

To emphasize this point, consider your responsibilities if the following circumstances occurred in your office:

1. A young husband, grieving his wife's sudden death, is told that cause of death is still undetermined pending lab results.
2. A 68-year-old widow is seen today by your physician after a sexual assault.

3. The owner of your town's only jewelry store is diagnosed with active tuberculosis. His quarantine requires that he close his store.

It will facilitate the inquiry and reporting of such situations and encourage the special care often required of patients if the physician's office has established policies regarding such matters. Each employee should know what kind of inquiry to make, how reporting is done, who is responsible, what information is required, and when and where the report is filed. A copy should always be kept for the office. It also is important to be aware of any community agencies that are available to provide information for the office and valuable services for the patients.

BIRTHS AND DEATHS

One important function of the physician is the recording of births and deaths. These certificates are legal documents, and as such, require truthfulness and prompt and proper completion. In some states, a criminal penalty will result if birth or death certificates are not properly completed. Some states refuse to accept certificates completed in inks other than black; others refuse to accept a certificate with any blanks.

The specific type of certificate required will vary from state to state. Generally, a stillbirth or fetal death, where the fetus has not passed the twentieth week of gestation, will not require a birth or death certificate.[1] In some states, however, a special stillbirth form is used; in others, it is necessary to file both a birth and death certificate. If the birth is considered a live birth and then the infant dies, both a standard birth and death certificate need to be completed.

In the event of a nonhospital birth, the person in attendance is responsible for initiating the birth certificate. In such a delivery, it is wise for a parent to verify that the process is completed within the designated time.

Check with your local health department, which furnishes the forms for birth and death certificates. A pamphlet entitled *Physicians' Handbook on Medical Certification: Death, Birth, and Fetal Death* by the U.S. Department of Health, Education and Welfare, Public Health Service, also is available upon request. The pamphlet provides detailed information for completing the standard forms. Figure 7 is an example of the Standard Certificate of Birth. Figure 8 is an example of the Standard Certificate of Death.

Generally speaking, physicians will sign a certificate giving the cause of death of the deceased upon whom they have been in professional attendance. Otherwise, someone of greater authority, such as the County Health Officer or Coroner, will assume the responsibility. In some states, a physician is forbidden by law to sign certain death certificates. Examples are a possible criminal death, death when the physician has not been in atten-

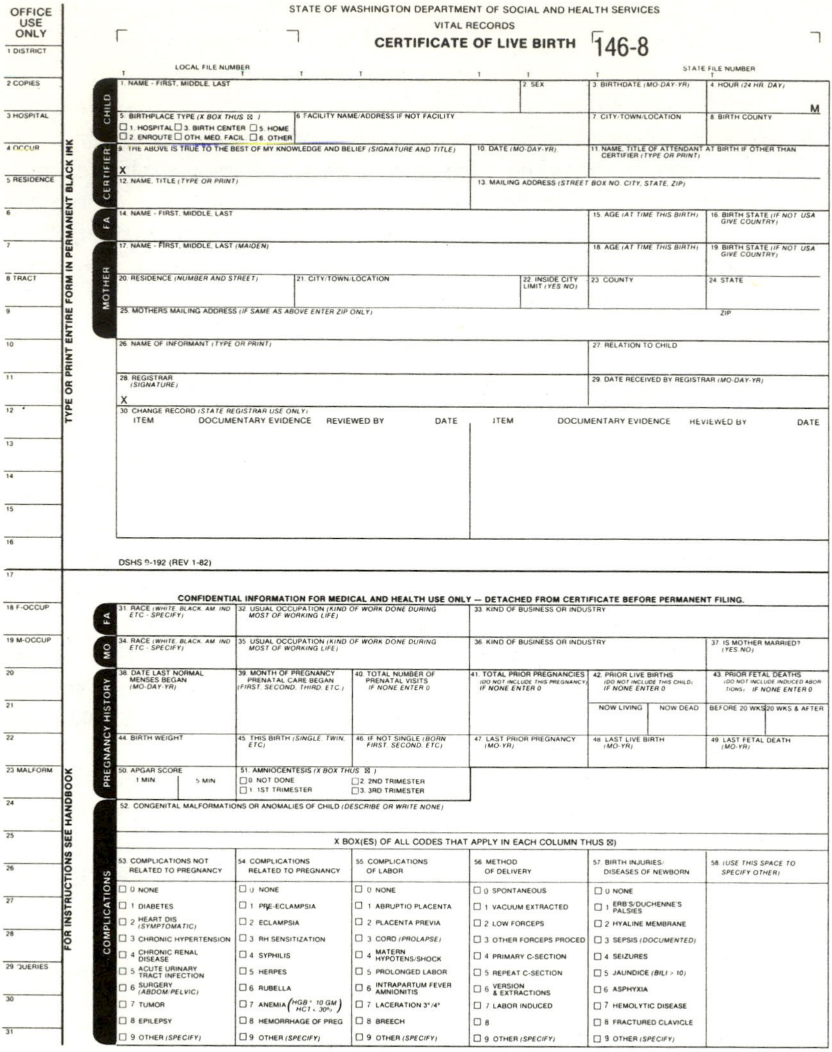

STATE OF WASHINGTON DEPARTMENT OF SOCIAL AND HEALTH SERVICES
VITAL RECORDS
CERTIFICATE OF LIVE BIRTH 146-8

OFFICE USE ONLY: 1 DISTRICT; 2 COPIES; 3 HOSPITAL; 4 OCCUR; 5 RESIDENCE; 6; 7; 8 TRACT; 9; 10; 11; 12; 13; 14; 15; 16; 17; 18 F-OCCUP; 19 M-OCCUP; 20; 21; 22; 23 MALFORM; 24; 25; 26; 27; 28; 29 QUERIES; 30; 31

TYPE OR PRINT ENTIRE FORM IN PERMANENT BLACK INK

LOCAL FILE NUMBER — STATE FILE NUMBER

CHILD: 1. NAME - FIRST, MIDDLE, LAST; 2 SEX; 3 BIRTHDATE (MO-DAY-YR); 4 HOUR (24 HR. DAY) M; 5 BIRTHPLACE TYPE (X BOX THUS ☒) ☐ 1. HOSPITAL ☐ 3. BIRTH CENTER ☐ 5. HOME ☐ 2. ENROUTE ☐ OTH. MED. FACIL. ☐ 6. OTHER; 6 FACILITY NAME/ADDRESS IF NOT FACILITY; 7 CITY/TOWN/LOCATION; 8 BIRTH COUNTY

CERTIFIER: 9. THE ABOVE IS TRUE TO THE BEST OF MY KNOWLEDGE AND BELIEF (SIGNATURE AND TITLE) X; 10 DATE (MO-DAY-YR); 11 NAME, TITLE OF ATTENDANT AT BIRTH IF OTHER THAN CERTIFIER (TYPE OR PRINT); 12 NAME, TITLE (TYPE OR PRINT); 13 MAILING ADDRESS (STREET BOX NO. CITY, STATE, ZIP)

FA: 14 NAME - FIRST, MIDDLE, LAST; 15 AGE (AT TIME THIS BIRTH); 16 BIRTH STATE (IF NOT USA GIVE COUNTRY)

MOTHER: 17 NAME - FIRST, MIDDLE, LAST (MAIDEN); 18 AGE (AT TIME THIS BIRTH); 19 BIRTH STATE (IF NOT USA GIVE COUNTRY); 20 RESIDENCE (NUMBER AND STREET); 21 CITY/TOWN/LOCATION; 22 INSIDE CITY LIMIT (YES NO); 23 COUNTY; 24 STATE; 25 MOTHERS MAILING ADDRESS (IF SAME AS ABOVE ENTER ZIP ONLY) ZIP

26 NAME OF INFORMANT (TYPE OR PRINT); 27 RELATION TO CHILD
28 REGISTRAR (SIGNATURE) X; 29 DATE RECEIVED BY REGISTRAR (MO-DAY-YR)
30 CHANGE RECORD (STATE REGISTRAR USE ONLY): ITEM | DOCUMENTARY EVIDENCE | REVIEWED BY | DATE | ITEM | DOCUMENTARY EVIDENCE | REVIEWED BY | DATE

DSHS 9-192 (REV 1-82)

CONFIDENTIAL INFORMATION FOR MEDICAL AND HEALTH USE ONLY — DETACHED FROM CERTIFICATE BEFORE PERMANENT FILING.

FOR INSTRUCTIONS SEE HANDBOOK

FA: 31 RACE (WHITE, BLACK, AM. IND. ETC.- SPECIFY); 32 USUAL OCCUPATION (KIND OF WORK DONE DURING MOST OF WORKING LIFE); 33 KIND OF BUSINESS OR INDUSTRY

MO: 34 RACE (WHITE, BLACK, AM. IND. ETC.- SPECIFY); 35 USUAL OCCUPATION (KIND OF WORK DONE DURING MOST OF WORKING LIFE); 36 KIND OF BUSINESS OR INDUSTRY; 37 IS MOTHER MARRIED? (YES NO)

PREGNANCY HISTORY: 38 DATE LAST NORMAL MENSES BEGAN (MO-DAY-YR); 39 MONTH OF PREGNANCY PRENATAL CARE BEGAN (FIRST, SECOND, THIRD, ETC.); 40 TOTAL NUMBER OF PRENATAL VISITS (IF NONE ENTER 0); 41 TOTAL PRIOR PREGNANCIES (DO NOT INCLUDE THIS PREGNANCY) (IF NONE ENTER 0); 42 PRIOR LIVE BIRTHS (DO NOT INCLUDE THIS CHILD) (IF NONE ENTER 0) NOW LIVING / NOW DEAD; 43 PRIOR FETAL DEATHS (DO NOT INCLUDE INDUCED ABORTIONS) (IF NONE ENTER 0) BEFORE 20 WKS / 20 WKS & AFTER; 44 BIRTH WEIGHT; 45 THIS BIRTH (SINGLE, TWIN, ETC.); 46 IF NOT SINGLE (BORN FIRST, SECOND, ETC.); 47 LAST PRIOR PREGNANCY (MO-YR); 48 LAST LIVE BIRTH (MO-YR); 49 LAST FETAL DEATH (MO-YR); 50 APGAR SCORE 1 MIN / 5 MIN; 51 AMNIOCENTESIS (X BOX THUS ☒) ☐ 0 NOT DONE ☐ 1 1ST TRIMESTER ☐ 2 2ND TRIMESTER ☐ 3 3RD TRIMESTER

COMPLICATIONS: 52 CONGENITAL MALFORMATIONS OR ANOMALIES OF CHILD (DESCRIBE OR WRITE NONE)

X BOX(ES) OF ALL CODES THAT APPLY IN EACH COLUMN THUS ☒

53 COMPLICATIONS NOT RELATED TO PREGNANCY	54 COMPLICATIONS RELATED TO PREGNANCY	55 COMPLICATIONS OF LABOR	56 METHOD OF DELIVERY	57 BIRTH INJURIES/ DISEASES OF NEWBORN	58 (USE THIS SPACE TO SPECIFY OTHER)
☐ 0 NONE	☐ 0 NONE	☐ 0 NONE	☐ 0 SPONTANEOUS	☐ 0 NONE	
☐ 1 DIABETES	☐ 1 PRE-ECLAMPSIA	☐ 1 ABRUPTIO PLACENTA	☐ 1 VACUUM EXTRACTED	☐ 1 ERB'S/DUCHENNE'S PALSIES	
☐ 2 HEART DIS (SYMPTOMATIC)	☐ 2 ECLAMPSIA	☐ 2 PLACENTA PREVIA	☐ 2 LOW FORCEPS	☐ 2 HYALINE MEMBRANE	
☐ 3 CHRONIC HYPERTENSION	☐ 3 RH SENSITIZATION	☐ 3 CORD (PROLAPSE)	☐ 3 OTHER FORCEPS PROCED	☐ 3 SEPSIS (DOCUMENTED)	
☐ 4 CHRONIC RENAL DISEASE	☐ 4 SYPHILIS	☐ 4 MATERN HYPOTENS/SHOCK	☐ 4 PRIMARY C-SECTION	☐ 4 SEIZURES	
☐ 5 ACUTE URINARY TRACT INFECTION	☐ 5 HERPES	☐ 5 PROLONGED LABOR	☐ 5 REPEAT C-SECTION	☐ 5 JAUNDICE (BILI > 10)	
☐ 6 SURGERY (ABDOM/PELVIC)	☐ 6 RUBELLA	☐ 6 INTRAPARTUM FEVER AMNIONITIS	☐ 6 VERSION & EXTRACTIONS	☐ 6 ASPHYXIA	
☐ 7 TUMOR	☐ 7 ANEMIA (HGB < 10 GM / HCT < 30%)	☐ 7 LACERATION 3°/4°	☐ 7 LABOR INDUCED	☐ 7 HEMOLYTIC DISEASE	
☐ 8 EPILEPSY	☐ 8 HEMORRHAGE OF PREG	☐ 8 BREECH	☐ 8	☐ 8 FRACTURED CLAVICLE	
☐ 9 OTHER (SPECIFY)	☐ 9 OTHER (SPECIFY)	☐ 9 OTHER (SPECIFY)	☐ 9 OTHER (SPECIFY)	☐ 9 OTHER (SPECIFY)	

FIGURE 7. Sample of birth certificate.

dance or is unable to determine the cause, and a violent or suspect death.[2] These cases are immediately turned over to a coroner, medical examiner, or an equivalent official for investigation and issuance of a death certificate.

Other circumstances that may require the reporting of death to the coroner are the occurrence of death within twenty-four hours after admission to a hospital or licensed health care facility, transporting the body out of state,[3] nonattendance by a physician during the three days prior to death, or death of an individual outside a hospital or licensed health care facility. The physician should not send the remains to a mortician without authorization from the next of kin or person responsible for funeral expenses.

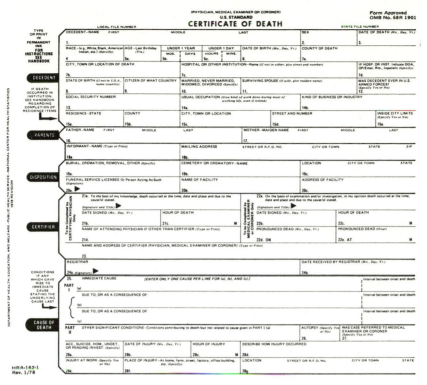

FIGURE 8. Sample of death certificate.

The urgency for prompt reporting by the physician is so the remains will not be disturbed and evidence will not be lost. This is particularly significant if an investigation and/or autopsy is to be performed. The physician may be the only one with access to facts that may determine (1) recognition of murder, (2) suspicion and/or prosecution of proper persons, (3) survivors' rights to insurance or other benefits, (4) death due to accidental violence or occupational hazard.[4]

As a courtesy to the family, it is imperative that the death certificate be completed and signed as quickly as possible so that funeral and financial arrangements can begin. Many states have a requirement that the death certificate be filed within 24 to 72 hours. The physician's office staff should realize that little can be done until the death certificate is signed.

COMMUNICABLE/NOTIFIABLE DISEASES

A disease is reportable when it concerns the public welfare and when it is a potentially pathological condition that may be transmitted directly or indirectly from one individual to another. The reporting of communicable diseases varies among states; however, local health departments publish lists of notifiable diseases (may be as many as 30 to 50) and the report format.

Physicians have the duty to report notifiable diseases by phone or mail. Reports are usually made by the office assistant, who telephones the county health department and furnishes the following information:

1. Disease (or suspected disease)
2. Name, address, age, and occupation of patient
3. Date of onset of disease
4. Name of person reporting.

To report by mail, use the appropriate case report cards furnished by the health department. Many diseases are reported on special forms. A check with your local health department may reveal as many as twenty or more specific forms for diseases. Some states encourage reporting by phone, with the statistical data being collected by the health department. Other states require the initial paperwork be completed at the time the notifiable disease is detected. Whatever method of reporting is used, be prompt, consistent, factual, and complete. Keep a copy of the report for the office files. The health department will attempt to determine the source of infection and mode of transmission so public health will be protected.

For more detailed information, consult your health department or the following two references: *Report of the Committee on Infectious Disease,* latest edition, American Academy of Pediatrics, P.O. Box 1034, Evanston, Illinois 60204; *Control of Communicable Diseases in Man,* latest edition, The American Public Health Association, 1015 Eighteenth Street, N.W., Washington, D.C. 20036.

REPORTABLE INJURIES

An injury is reportable when it concerns the public welfare and requires reporting to the proper authority; for example, injuries resulting from gun or knife wounds. Some states have detailed requirements for reporting injuries. Others have none. Check with the local and state medical associations and law enforcement agencies for specific information.

Generally, injuries caused by lethal weapons, such as guns and knives, are reported, and patients are treated in emergency or hospital facilities. When possible rape victims or battered persons seek treatment from private physicians, patients may be treated in the office or immediately referred to the emergency room of a local hospital.

In urban areas there may be community service agencies such as "Rape Relief" or "Sexual Assault Centers." The physician may refer the patient to such an agency for additional, unique specialized services offered to the victim. However, if these services are not available or the patient chooses to be treated by the physician alone, the physician needs information from law enforcement agencies regarding the reporting, obtaining, securing, and handling of medicolegal evidence.

It is important to treat the patient as soon as possible after the injury or assault, not only for the patient's welfare but also to preserve evidence of possible criminal acts. Rape victims particularly need to feel supported, cared for, and to feel that the violent act will make no difference in how they are treated by people.

CHILD ABUSE

According to the Council for the Prevention of Child Abuse and Neglect, child abuse is the second largest cause of death in children under five.[5] Incidents of child abuse and neglect may be seen in a hospital or a physician's office when a child displays fractures, burns, severe bruises, and questionable injuries. Not so obvious injuries may include dislocations, cerebrospinal trauma, and internal injuries resulting from blows to the abdomen. Malnutrition, poor growth pattern, poor hygiene, gross dental problems, and unattended medical needs[6] also may indicate neglect and/or abuse.

Currently, each state has statutes or laws defining child abuse and mandating that suspected child abuse and neglect be reported. Any person who has reasonable cause to suspect that a child may be the victim of abuse or neglect may report, in good faith, to law enforcement and/or child protection agencies. Such persons are protected against liability as a result of making the report provided there is reasonable cause to suspect child abuse or neglect.

Some states *require* that certain individuals report suspected abuse and neglect. These include health professionals, social service personnel, law enforcement personnel, educators, and any professional person working with children.[7] Some states also allow a hospital administrator or a physician to detain a child legally without a guardian's consent in such instances.

The function of reporting is to identify incidents of *suspected* abuse and neglect, not to *prove* abuse or neglect. Failure to report suspected abuse or neglect may result in civil or criminal penalties.

The report may be oral or written or both. Immediate reporting is paramount so a proper investigation can be initiated.

Information required in the report may include the following:[8]

1. Name, address, and age of child.
2. Name and address of child's parents (or guardians).
3. Nature and extent of the injury, neglect or abuse.
4. Any evidence of previous incidents of abuse or neglect, including their nature and extent.
5. Any other information that may be helpful in establishing the cause of the child's injuries, neglect, or death, and the identity of the perpetrator(s).

If a crime has been committed, law enforcement must be notified.

Child abuse and neglect are difficult problems, not easily solved. While laws were meant to protect the welfare of the child, they may, in fact, safeguard the family unit more. However, it is important for physicians and employees to be advocates of the child's well-being and nonjudgmental of parents.

DRUG ABUSE

Drug misuse or abuse is found in every sector of society. It occurs increasingly in affluent suburbs as well as in the slums. It is becoming commonplace in schools and industry.[9] Pharmacists are receiving fake telephone prescription orders. Physicians are being pestered by abusers seeking controlled substances for their own personal use or their resale in the streets. There are few statutes or regulatory requirements related to drug abuse, other than the Controlled Substances Act discussed in Chapter 4. However, physicians and their employees have a public duty to be alert to this problem and do everything possible to prevent its increase.

A common problem is a drug abuser securing the same prescription drug from more than one physician and pharmacy in an area. Often abusers go from "door to door" of medical clinics and offices with a convincing tale of woe or set of symptoms that may warrant a prescription drug. The office assistant often will be convinced by the abuser(s) that this is a valid complaint and may be coerced into becoming an advocate for the abuser. Another problem occurs when some physicians become what are known as "script doctors." They freely and excessively prescribe potentially dangerous drugs.

The American Medical Association (AMA), in a report of the Council on Scientific Affairs, recommends that pharmacists and physicians cooperate at the national, state, and local levels to curtail prescription drug abuse and to promote appropriate prescribing practices by physicians.[10]

Some communities have established "hot lines" so that descriptions of suspected drug abusers and their mode of operation can be communicated to physicians and pharmacists in the area. One technique that works well is for the assistant or physician to ask for a positive picture identification card of each new patient. Most abusers will not produce such identification. It is also wise for an assistant to be advised that the physician will authorize no prescriptions without first seeing the patient.

Physicians and office staff are encouraged to treat prescription blanks with the same security they treat their checkbooks.[11] It is best not to keep controlled substances on the premises if at all possible. Any that are kept must be under lock and key and immediately reported if stolen or lost. Be alert to the regular patient who may be seeing more than one doctor for the same complaint and receiving several prescriptions by carefully questioning of patients during examination. Pharmacists watch closely for this problem, but the number of pharmacies in large cities makes effective control nearly impossible.

The market for prescription drugs on the street is a lucrative one. Dilaudid tablets will sell for $60 to $70 each, with Meprobamate, Darvon, Librium, and Valium bringing from $5 to $15 each.[12] In these times, it is particularly important that physicians and health professionals establish firm and clear office procedures to curb the increase of drug misuse and abuse.

REFERENCES

1. MORITZ, AA AND MORRIS, RC: *Handbook of Legal Medicine.* CV Mosby, St Louis, 1970, p 199.

2. IBID, p 200.

3. IBID, p 4.

4. IBID, p 10.

5. MILLS, DD: *CPS indicated: 'It's understaffed, underpaid, underqualified.'* The Seattle *Times,* August 2, 1981, E-1.

6. MCKITTRICK, CA: *Child abuse: Recognition and reporting by health professionals. The Nursing Clinics of North America* 16:1. March 1981, p. 107.

7. DREITZER, M: *Legal aspects of child abuse. The Nursing Clinics of North America* 16:1. March 1981, p 149.

8. WASHINGTON STATE DEPARTMENT OF SOCIAL AND HEALTH SERVICES: *Protecting the Abused and Neglected Child.* Department of Social and Health Services, Olympia, WA, 22-163 (4/80).

9. TEBROCK, HE, MD: *Drug Abuse and Misuse.* US Government Printing Office, Drug Enforcement Administration, US Department of Justice, 1979, p 1.

10. AMERICAN PHARMACEUTICAL ASSOCIATION: *AMA urges cooperation in Rx drug abuse fight. Apharmacy Weekly* 20:24, Bremerton, WA, 1981, p 99.

11. *Pharmacists request . . . Bulletin of the Kitsap County Medical Society,* Vol 17, Bremerton, WA, May-June 1981, p 2.

12. IBID.

DISCUSSION QUESTIONS

1. In the three examples at the beginning of the chapter (pp. 52-53), discuss your responsibilities in each situation, possible referral agencies available, and possible problems encountered. How can you be of assistance to your physician-employer?

2. What problems occur when a death certificate remains unsigned?

3. What are the future implications if a birth is not reported?

4. Explore possible referral agencies in your community and share your findings.

5. Dramatize different drug abusers who may frequent a medical office. How can office personnel be alert to these abusers?

CHAPTER 6

THE MEDICAL OFFICE IN LITIGATION

LEARNING OBJECTIVES

Upon successful completion of this chapter, you will:

1. Explain three circumstances that may involve physicians in litigation.

2. List three elements necessary for a contract to be valid.

3. Identify the Four D's of Negligence for physicians.

4. Define tort and give three examples common to the medical office.

5. Define Statute of Limitations and identify the three most common points for the Statute of Limitations to begin.

6. List two similarities and dissimilarities between subpoena and *subpoena duces tecum.*

7. Name two circumstances calling for an expert witness.

DEFINITIONS

Breach of Contract. A failure to comply with the terms of a valid contract.

Defamation. Spoken or written words concerning someone that tend to injure that person's reputation and for which damages can be recovered. Two types of defamation include: a) *libel:* defamatory writing; published material such as writing, effigy, or picture; b) *slander:* malicious defamatory spoken word.

Deposition. A written record of oral testimony made before a public officer for use in a lawsuit.

Expert Witness (medical). Person trained in medicine who can testify in a court of law as to what the professional standard of care is in the same or similar communities.

Res Ipsa Loquitur. A Latin phrase, "the thing speaks for itself." A doctrine of negligence law.

Statute. A law enacted by a legislative body of the state or Federal government.

Subpoena duces tecum. A court order requiring a witness to appear and bring certain records or tangible items to a trial or deposition.

Summons. A court order to appear as a defendant in a complaint.

Tort. Wrongful act committed by one person or against another person or property that does not arise as the result of a breach of contract.

INTRODUCTION

One of the greatest fears of employees and their physicians in the medical office is the threat of litigation. Caring for persons who may be ill, apprehensive, in pain, or may be suffering from a terminal condition is risky. Such a risk carries the possibility of litigation and becomes a reality when a summons is served at the medical office on the physician or when someone is subpoenaed to testify.

There are many reasons why litigation may be sought. A patient may sue the physician for negligence. Perhaps a contractual arrangement has been violated, a tort has been committed or legal evidence is needed by the court. The statute of limitations regarding timeliness, how subpoenas are to be handled, and what is expected of an expert witness are all important concerns for medical office employees and their physicians.

LIABILITY

Liability can be either civil or criminal. Criminal liability is less common in the medical office than civil liability.

CRIMINAL LIABILITY

Criminal liability results when an individual commits an act that is considered to be an offense against society as a whole.

Examples of criminal liability for the physician include performing an act of active euthanasia and the evasion or breach of the narcotics laws.

Also, physicians found to be grossly negligent or ignorant in the death of a patient may be held criminally responsible. In some states, the failure of physicians to make certain reports (for example, child abuse) required by law may result in criminal prosecution.[1]

CIVIL LIABILITY

Physicians must use ordinary and reasonable skill commonly held by other reputable practitioners when caring for patients. Failure to perform professional duties competently is *negligence* as discussed in the last chapter. Physicians should always perform in the realm of safety and secure all necessary data on which to base a sound judgment. Physicians are expected to exhaust all possible resources available to them when treating their patients. This will include obtaining a thorough medical history, a complete physical examination, and necessary laboratory tests.

Res Ipsa Loquitur

The doctrine of *res ipsa loquitur,* "the thing speaks for itself," is a rule of the law of negligence. It relates chiefly to cases of (1) foreign bodies and slipping instruments in surgical procedures, (2) burns from heating modalities, and (3) injury to a portion of the patient's body outside the field of treatment. In other words, the negligence is obvious; the result was such that it could not have occurred without someone being negligent.

Abandonment

Once the physician-patient relationship has been established, physicians can be found liable if they abandon their patients. The only provision here is for the physician to withdraw formally from the case or discharge the patient formally. This requires giving reasonable notice to the patient and ample time for the patient to secure another physician. This should be done in writing with a copy for the files.

A physician may wish to withdraw from the case if the patient fails to follow instructions or take the prescribed medications, or does not return for recommended appointments. To withdraw formally from a case, a physician should notify the patient in writing, state the reasons for the dismissal, and indicate a future date at which the physician is no longer responsible. It is wise to send such a letter by certified mail with a return receipt requested. A copy of the letter and the returned receipt are kept in the patient's file. To further protect a physician from abandoning a patient, all canceled and missed appointments should be noted in the patient's chart.

Confidentiality

Physicians must keep confidential any communication from the patient necessary to provide treatment unless otherwise required by law. The patient's privacy must be protected. Physicians and their employees must be extremely careful that all information gained through the care of the patient is kept confidential. Care should be taken so that any information about a patient cannot be overheard by others.

Privilege forbids physicians from revealing information about patients in court. Privilege belongs to the patient rather than the physician. If a patient waives privilege, the physician may not withhold testimony. Not all states recognize the patient-physician communication as privileged. The court will determine if the importance of the evidence outweighs any damage caused by disclosure of the information.

Contracts

Medical office employees and their physicians are parties to contracts on a daily basis. When a physician accepts a patient, a contract has been made. When the office assistant calls an office supply company to reorder office stationery, the assistant acts as the physician's agent in making a contract. For contracts to be valid, the following must exist. There must be (1) an agreement between two or more competent persons (2) upon consideration or payment (3) to do or not to do a task that is legal.[2]

In other words, the contract must be an understanding between two or more people to do or not to do a certain task for payment or the rendering of a benefit, and the agreement must be lawful. An example in the medical office occurs when a patient calls the office to make an appointment for an annual physical examination. The appointment is kept and the physician gives the examination. Assuming that the physician is a bona-fide physician and the patient is a competent adult, parts one and two of the contract exist. The performance of a physical examination is a lawful act, so part three of the contract exists. The patient is given a statement of the charges, and the fee is paid. Hence the contract is valid in all respects.

A contract can be expressed or implied. An expressed contract can be written or oral, but all facets of the contract must be specifically stated and understood. A written contract requires that all aspects of the agreement be in writing. Each state in its Statute of Frauds identifies those contracts that must be in writing. Usually included in this list are deeds and mortgages. These statutes, though they differ from state to state, come from the original English Statute of Frauds of 1677.[3] A section from the original statute that is pertinent to the medical office is that an agreement made by a third party to pay for the medical expenses of another has to be in writing to be valid. If Elaine tells the medical receptionist that she will pay the medical expenses of her good friend Diane, the receptionist should ask Elaine to fill out a form to that effect and affix her signature to it.

Implied contracts are the most common form in the medical office. Such contracts occur every time the physician and patient discuss what course of treatment to take and an agreement is reached. An implied agreement does not provide for a specific expression of the parties involved, but is still valid if all points of the contract exist. An implied contract may be implied from the facts of circumstances of the situation or by the law. When a patient complains of a sore throat and the physician does a throat culture to diagnose and treat the ailment, a contract is implied by the circumstances of the situation. A contract implied by the law is seen in the example of the physician who administers epinephrine when a patient goes into anaphylactic shock in the examination room. The law will say that the physician did what the patient would have requested had there been an expressed agreement.

Contracts made by the mentally incompetent, the legally insane, those under heavy influence of drugs or alcohol, infants, and some minors are not valid. Such persons are not considered to be competent by the law.

Medical office employees are generally considered "agents" of their physician-employers. An agent is a person appointed by a principal party to perform authorized acts in the name and under the control and direction of the principal. In this position, medical office employees must be careful of their actions that may become binding on their physician. For example, an employee may "promise a cure" when, in fact, it may not be possible.

Four D's of Negligence

The Committee on Medicolegal Problems of the American Medical Association, in a 1963 report, stated:

> To obtain a judgment against a physician for negligence, the patient must present evidence of what have been referred to as the "four D's." The patient must show: (1) that the physician owed a *duty* to the patient, (2) that the physician was *derelict* and breached that duty by failing to act as the ordinary, competent physician in the same community would have acted under the same or similar circumstances, (3) that such failure or breach was the *direct cause* of the patient's injuries, and (4) that *damages* to the patient resulted therefrom.[4]

Duty exists when the physician-patient relationship has been established. For example, the patient calls the office to make an appointment, keeps the appointment, and makes another to return for further treatment.

Derelict is more difficult to define. The patient must prove that the physician failed to comply with the duty required and dictated by the situation.

Direct cause implies that any damages or injuries that resulted from the physician's breach of duty were directly related to that breach and that no intermittent circumstances or intervening causes could have caused the damages.

Damages refer to the injuries suffered by the patient. The most common in medical professional liability cases is *compensatory* damage, which may be *general* or *special*.

Compensation for *general* damages usually provides compensation for injuries or losses that are natural and necessary consequences of the physician's neglect (for example, compensation for pain and suffering, loss of bodily members). Losses must be proved; monetary loss need not be.

Special compensation is for injuries or losses not necessarily a consequence of the physician's neglect (for example, cost of medical and hospital care, loss of earnings). Both injuries or losses *and* monetary value must be proved.[5]

Torts

Medical office employees or their physicians may commit a tort that may result in litigation. A tort is a wrongful act committed by one person or against another person or property that does not arise as the result of a breach of contract. There must be (1) damage to the patient, proximately caused by (2) conduct of the physician (or employee) that falls below (3) the standard of care governing the physician (or employee)[6] (Four D's of Negligence). If a physician commits a wrongful act against a patient with no resultant patient harm, a tort has not been committed.

There are two main classifications of torts—*intentional* and *negligent* wrongs. Intentional wrongs involve the *intentional* commission of a violation of another person's rights. Negligent wrongs are not intentional and may be the result of the *omission* as well as the *commission* of an act.

The physician who commits a tort is liable for damages in a civil action, rather than a criminal one. The plaintiff may, in a civil suit, seek compensation from the physician for damages suffered. The wrongful act itself, however, may end up in both criminal court and civil court, but there will be separate trials, that is, one civil and the other criminal. Recall from Chapter 1 that in a civil case the plaintiffs have to show, by a preponderance of evidence, that a tort has been committed, whereas in a criminal case, the prosecution must prove its case beyond a reasonable doubt.

Some of the more common tort examples likely to occur in the medical office include (1) battery, (2) defamation, and (3) invasion of privacy.

1. *Battery:* unlawful touching, beating, or laying hold of persons or their clothing without consent. When a battery occurs, it is an

individual's right that has been invaded. Individuals have the right to be free from invasion of their person. It makes no difference whether or not the procedure constituting the battery improves the patient's health. The patient has to consent to the touching.

Example: An 18-year-old with a severely injured arm comes into the medical office. The physician cuts off the tan leather jacket as the patient cries, "I told you not to ruin my jacket. It cost me two paychecks!"

2. *Defamation:* spoken/written words that tend to injure a person's reputation and for which damages can be recovered. Two types include (a) libel and (b) slander.
    a. *libel:* malicious defamatory writing; any published material, for example, writing, effigy, picture.
    b. *slander:* false or malicious defamatory spoken word.

For defamation to be a tort, a third person must hear or see the slander or libel and understand it.

Example: A patient in the reception area overhears a telephone conversation, reporting a positive test for venereal disease to an individual who is recognized as the mayor. The patient remarks to another patient in the room, "Did you hear that? The mayor has VD!"

3. *Invasion of Privacy:* unauthorized publicity of patient information. Medical records and/or treatments cannot be released without the patient's knowledge and permission. Patients have the right to be left alone, the right to be free from unwanted publicity and exposure to public view.

Example: An instructor shows photographs of a patient's unusual disease/condition to a class without authorization.

Example: An office employee permits a part of a medical record of a 50-year-old patient who gave birth to triplets to be published by the local newspaper without authorization because "it is so unusual."

Torts can be prevented by practicing legally and ethically above reproach. The standard of care in medical offices needs to be excellent. The privacy of patients must be guarded, their bodies and possessions must be respected, and their reputations must be protected. The rights of patients are to be protected by all who come in contact with them.

STATUTE OF LIMITATIONS

State legislatures have established *statutes of limitations* that restrict the time allowed for individuals to initiate any type of legal action. There is great variation from state to state regarding the length of time allowed for starting a lawsuit. The time limit is generally from one to six years.

Waltz and Inbau[7] in *Medical Jurisprudence* identify the three most common points when medical malpractice action of the statute of limitations may begin. They are: "(1) the time when the negligent act was allegedly committed, (2) the time when the resultant injury was discovered or should have been discovered had the patient acted with reasonable alertness, and (3) the time when the doctor-patient relationship or the treatments, if there was a continuous series of them, ended."

It is wise to understand your state's law on the subject as well as how it has been interpreted. There usually will be a separate statute of limitations for tort actions and for contracts.

Circumstances that may alter the statute of limitations occur with a person who is legally insane or has not yet reached the age of majority. Therefore, a person declared legally insane will not come under the statute of limitations until the period of insanity has ended. And in the case of pediatricians, the time period in the statute may not apply until the child has reached the age of majority—usually 18.

Physicians and their employees must concern themselves with the statute of limitations when considering the retention of their medical records as well as when they could be involved in a malpractice suit. Legal counsel should be sought for interpretation and advice.

SUBPOENAS

Physicians may find themselves in court even though they and their employees have practiced good preventive measures. No matter what the dispute or reason for litigation, physicians need to be adequately prepared. The reasons for court appearances are numerous, but most frequently the physician will be a defendant or a witness in criminal trials, insanity and probate contests, personal injury actions, or cases arising under life, health, or accident insurance policies.[8]

In any of these cases, physicians may appear with or without a subpoena. A subpoena is a court order commanding attendance in a specific court or office, at a specific time, under penalty for failure to do so. The subpoena may be signed by the clerk of court, a notary public, or an attorney. The subpoena may require a deposition to be taken rather than actual appearance in court.

The attendance requested in a subpoena may be of a person (physician) and/or of data (medical record). The latter is a *subpoena duces tecum,* which requires the witness to appear and to bring certain records. The physician most likely would not need to appear to identify a record, as proper identification can usually be done by an employee.

Whatever the type of subpoena, it must be served within the state issued, in person to the one named on the subpoena, and it may authorize witness fees and/or mileage fees. If the physician is being subpoenaed, it must be hand-delivered to the physician. If the record is subpoenaed, it may be served to an employee. Any time you have questions about a subpoena or its circumstances, contact your attorney immediately.

EXPERT WITNESS

In medical cases, an expert witness is a person trained in medicine who can testify in court as to what the professional standard of care is in the same or similar community. An expert witness is necessary if the subject of the court action is beyond the general understanding of the average layperson or if the knowledge of the expert witness will aid in discovering the truth.

As expert witnesses, physicians testify as to what they see, hear, and know to be fact. Opinions, hearsay, and conclusions are not admissible;[9] however, in most states experts are allowed to form an opinion based on their experience and expertise. Expert witnesses in medical cases are usually skilled in the art, science, or profession of medicine and may be practicing medicine or teaching in a school of medicine. They are expected to be reputable, honest, and impartial. The attorneys will try to establish the witness's training, experience, intelligence and accuracy. Witnesses should talk in lay terms, rather than medical language, bearing in mind their dress and appearance may influence the judge and jury. Attorneys cannot prompt or cue witnesses.

Expert witnesses may wish to illustrate or clarify their testimony by employing photographs, maps, diagrams, charts, roentgenograms, skeletons, and models.[10] In some instances, sketch artists or illustrators may be employed. However, any materials used need the proper foundation and cerification established in court by attorneys. Seeing may be more believable. During cross-examination, witnesses may face difficulty. Attorneys may try to intimidate, or create confusion. Witnesses should take their time and answer truthfully. They should not be afraid to say, "I don't know," if that is the case.

Expert witnesses are entitled to a fee commensurate with their time, preparation, and participation in the case.[11] If questioned during cross-examination regarding a fee for witnessing, answer truthfully. A fee should be established prior to serving as an expert witness rather than on a contingency basis.

If you or your physician-employer is subpoenaed to be an expert witness, it is an excellent idea to seek legal counsel. An attorney will guide, advise, and take whatever legal action is indicated for you. A good reference book is *Testifying in Court: The Advanced Course* by Jack E. Horsley with John Carlova, Medical Economics Company, 1975.

Although it has been said several times already, it cannot be over-stressed how important legal counsel is if there are any questions or doubts. Physicians often seek consultations on difficult medical problems and should do no less for themselves and their employees if faced with litigation.

EVIDENCE

Gathering of evidence is more likely to occur in the emergency room or hospital setting. There will be situations, however, in the medical office where employees and physicians need to be knowledgeable of methods of proper collection and preservation of evidence. When in doubt, seek professional guidance from attorneys and proper authorities.

In the medical office, physicians may gather legal evidence knowingly or unknowingly. Later they may be asked to offer the evidence or will be subpoenaed to give the evidence. Some common office situations may include the female toddler's urinalysis showing sperm, the young male seeking medical treatment because he has been sexually assaulted, or a patient entering with a superficial knife wound. Circumstances just described may involve physicians as witnesses in litigation where proper examination and documentation are essential.

One of the first ways evidence is documented is through medical records. A frequent reason for losing a malpractice lawsuit, perhaps for a large settlement, is improper documentation in medical records. Specifically, physicians must record the time of patient arrival, and a complete explanation of the patient's condition, both physically and emotionally. Obviously, treatment of the patient is paramount, but documentation must follow. Interpretation in the records of the findings may be risky.[12]

Evidence may be in the form of a complete written description, roentgenograms, photographs, clothing, samples for laboratory testing, or samples of foreign objects. Roentgenograms and photographs need to be dated and labeled with the patient's name. Photographs may need a brief description. Both roentgenograms and photographs should be stored in envelopes to protect them. Any objects and clothing should be properly and carefully removed, and labeled. It is best not to cut clothing unless necessary and then along seams. Handle objects as little as possible to avoid damaging them.[13] Any body fluids, such as vomitus or gastric washings, should be saved, especially in poisoning cases, for future analysis.

You may be requested by law enforcement to take patient samples such as blood, vaginal, oral or rectal smears, fingernail or hair clippings.[14] They, too, must be properly labeled and preserved. Every piece of evidence needs to be preserved as much as possible and securely stored in a locked place to avoid tampering or loss.

It is a good idea to have only one employee handle all evidence, thus preventing it from becoming inadmissible because it cannot be properly traced or verified. When giving evidence to the proper authorities, ask for a receipt for your office files.

Physicians should cooperate when law enforcement authorities need to talk to the patient. The physician should be neither overprotective of the patient, nor should the patient be jeopardized. The sooner authorities receive information from the patient, however, the quicker they can begin their investigation.[15]

When the patient dies in the office or arrives dead, it is wise to call the medical examiner or coroner immediately and avoid any touching or moving of the remains. To protect any possible evidence, it is best not to remove any tubes or paraphernalia from the patient.[16]

SUMMARY

Much additional information could be added to the topics in this chapter; each area is a book all its own. The data included should be sufficient to assist physicians and medical office employees to keep their offices out of litigation. If office litigation becomes a reality, however, seek professional legal advice promptly.

REFERENCES

1. MORITZ, AA AND MORRIS, RC: *Handbook of Legal Medicine*, ed 3. WB Saunders, Philadelphia, 1975, p 147.

2. SARNER, J: *The Nurse and the Law*. WB Saunders, Philadelphia, 1981, p 113.

3. FARMER, RA ET AL: *What You Should Know About Contracts*. ARCO Publishing, New York, 1969, p 56.

4. FREDERICK, PM AND KINN, MD: *The Medical Office Assistant*. WB Saunders, Philadelphia, 1981, p 52.

5. IBID.

6. WALTZ, JR, INBAU, FF ET AL: *Medical Jurisprudence*. Macmillan, New York, 1971, p 41.

7. IBID, p 135.

8. MORITZ, p 184.

9. STREIFF, CJ AND THE HEALTH LAW CENTER (EDS): *Nursing and the Law*. Aspen Systems Corporation, Rockville, MD, 1975, p 137.

10. MORITZ, p 185.

11. STREIFF, p 103.

12. WALTZ, p 330.

13. IBID, p 339.

14. IBID, p 342.

15. IBID, p 353.

16. IBID, p 351.

DISCUSSION QUESTIONS

1. For each area of liability discussed in the chapter, give an example which might occur in the medical office.

2. Contrast and compare a tort and a breach of contract. Give an example of each.

3. Cite two examples of torts a medical office employee could commit.

4. There generally are three methods to determine when the Statute of Limitations on medical malpractice action may begin. What are they?

5. When might an expert witness be needed? What suggestions might you have for the witness's court preparation and appearance?

6. The physician gives you an envelope of x-rays and a sealed bag of clothing items, asking you to keep these safe until law enforcement officials arrive. How would you keep them safe? Why is this important?

CHAPTER 7

CONSENT

LEARNING OBJECTIVES

Upon successful completion of this chapter, you will:

1. Define consent, and explain, in your own words, why consent is important.

2. Give an example of (a) verbal consent, (b) nonverbal consent, and (c) written consent.

3. Compare informed and uninformed consent.

4. List the four elements of the Doctrine of Informed Consent.

5. Identify special situations in consent:
   a. minors
   b. spouses
   c. language barriers
   d. when consent is not necessary

6. Discuss the role of the office employee in obtaining consent.

DEFINITIONS

Consent. The affirmation by a patient to allow touching, examination, and/or treatment by medically authorized personnel.

Doctrine of Informed Consent. Specific guidelines for consent, usually identified by medical practice acts at the state level.

Informed Consent. The patient's right to know before agreeing to a procedure. The patient not only gives permission to allow touching, examination, and/or treatment by medically authorized personnel, but also understands what has been consented to.

Minor. A person who has not reached the age of majority. The age of majority is usually 18 years.

   Emancipated Minor. A person under 18 years of age who is free of parental care.

Uninformed Consent. Patient gives permission to allow touching, examination, and/or treatment by medically authorized personnel, but really *does not* understand what has been consented to.

INTRODUCTION

All medical office employees at one time or another may be involved in the consent process with patients. While it is the primary responsibility of the health care provider to inform the patient of proposed treatment in order to obtain consent for a procedure, it is not uncommon for a patient to ask questions of any of the employees. Consequently, it is important that everyone understand all aspects of consent.

DEFINITION

Consent is the affirmation by a patient to allow touching, examination, and/or treatment by medically authorized personnel. Consent allows patients to determine what will be done with their bodies. Without consent, intentional touching can be considered a criminal offense. Consent is authorization given by implications of (1) a patient's behavior, (2) a medical contract, or (3) by law. Consent is obtained through word or action. Consent may be given orally, expressed by nonverbal behavior, or expressed in writing. Consider the following examples:

   Example 1. A patient calls complaining of a persistent, productive cough. When the receptionist makes the appointment with the physician, the patient has given consent for examination, which may include throat examination and culture.

   Example 2. When the physician requires a blood test for diagnosis, and the patient comes to the lab with a rolled-up sleeve, the patient is giving consent.

   Example 3. A patient is scheduled for an office surgical procedure and signs an appropriate consent form. This action constitutes a medical contract between the patient and the physician. Written consent has been obtained.

   Example 4. If a patient who comes to the office suddenly stops breathing during the physician's examination, the physician will take immediate action to restore breathing and prevent any further damage. Consent is implied by law in an emergency situation when a patient is unable to give consent. An emergency is said to exist when there is immediate danger to the patient and action is necessary to save the patient's life or prevent further damage.

Integral to consent is the patient's belief that the person to whom consent is given has the knowledge, skill, and ability to perform such tasks. In our examples, the patient has a right to expect that the physician has the ability to determine the need for a throat culture, perform the required surgery, and administer emergency treatment. Likewise, the patient can expect the lab technician to know proper venipuncture techniques.

INFORMED / UNINFORMED CONSENT

The ideal is that all consent is "informed," with the patient understanding all facets of the consent. Patients who are a party to consent are usually informed or have sufficient understanding of the circumstances surrounding their consent. "Uninformed" consent occurs when the patient gives permission but really does not understand or comprehend what has been consented to.

There are many occasions arising in the medical office that involve complicated medical procedures, often difficult for patients to understand. Informed consent is important to give the physician permission to act. To insure that proper consent is obtained, it is usually put in writing. States have specific guidelines usually established in The Doctrine of Informed Consent.

THE DOCTRINE OF INFORMED CONSENT

Written consent is intentional and deliberate. The essential elements of The Docrine of Informed Consent will almost always mandate that it be in writing. Informed consent is the patient's right to know before agreeing to a procedure.

The necessary elements require that the patient understand the nature of the illness and be told in language easily understood:

1. What the procedure is and how it is to be performed.
2. Possible risks involved as well as expected results.
3. Any alternative procedures or treatments and their risks.
4. Results if no treatment is given.

To further illustrate the necessary elements in informed consent, consider the following example:

Phil, age 65, has been diagnosed by the physician as having adenocarcinoma. His physician is careful to explain the nature of this particular disease to Phil and its possible progression in his body. The physician then outlines the possible forms of treatment, such as surgery, chemotherapy, or radiation, being careful to explain the risks of each as well as possible outcomes. It is not uncommon for the physician to encourage a particular form of treatment even before the patient asks for a recommendation. Here the physician has knowledge of Phil's particular case that may be expected to give credence to such a recommendation. However, the physician should be careful to also explain the possible risks of no treatment at all. While the patient looks to the physician for medical information and recommendations, the decision will be the patient's alone.

In Phil's situation, as with most others, all office staff members must be sensitive to the impact of such a decision. For consent to be meaningful, Phil may need time to comprehend the essential elements of the consent. This may include talking with family members, seeking a second opinion, considering financial implications, or just being alone. Staff members also need to be prepared to clarify, further explain, or direct additional questions to the physician if the patient so indicates. Not until a later time will the actual written consent be finalized and the physician be able to proceed. The written consent must reflect each of the elements described and also should contain the patient's signature, the physician's signature, and the signature of a witness.

PROBLEMS IN CONSENT

Consent may be difficult to obtain in treatment of a *minor,* a person who has not reached the age of majority. Generally, the age of majority is 18 years; however, it may vary. In most states a minor is unable to give consent for medical care *except* in special cases when a minor is married, pregnant, emancipated, suspected of having venereal disease or possible problems in drug or alcohol abuse, or is in need of psychiatric care. In all other situations, the physician or staff should attempt to reach parents and/ or legal guardians for consent.

Legal implications to consider when treating a minor are:

1. A minor has the right to confidentiality. A 16-year-old who seeks a prescription for birth control pills has the right for that information to be kept confidential.
2. A minor who may legally consent to treatment may not be financially responsible. If the 16-year-old in the first example does not pay when services are given, it may be difficult to collect from parents who have not given their consent.
3. A minor's legal guardian may have to be determined—a special problem in the case of divorce and remarriage. If the father of a

child is financially responsible, but the child resides with the mother, who may properly consent for treatment?

It is imperative to be knowledgeable regarding your own state consent laws and have your attorney's recommendations when problems occur.

While the law that governs consent may be well defined when dealing with minors, it may be very vague or even nonexistent with respect to *spouses.* Heightened consciousness of the rights of women has made significant impact on the legal system. Certainly, more can be expected in the future.

It is generally recognized that a spouse has the right to consent to and receive medical care and treatment without a spouse's approval. However, there are some situations when medical providers will seek consent from husband and wife as an additional precautionary measure. Such situations include convenience sterilization and abortion.

Other problems in consent may arise in the case of *foster children, stroke patients* who cannot communicate, the *mentally incompetent, senile persons,* and those temporarily or permanently *under the influence of drugs or alcohol.* A legal guardian who can give consent may have to be appointed by the courts. It is imperative for the medical office staff to determine who is legally responsible in each case. In any event, however, when there is immediate danger to life or limb, the law implies consent for treatment for these individuals without consent from the responsible party.

With increased immigration in this country, *language* can be a barrier to informed consent. An interpreter may be necessary so information for consent may be given in the native tongue.

There are a number of exceptions to informed consent peculiar to each state. Such examples may include:

1. The physician may not need to disclose risks commonly known.
2. The physician may not be responsible for failing to disclose risk(s) when the knowledge might be detrimental to the patient's best interest.
3. A physician may not need to disclose risks if the patient requests to remain ignorant.

A patient has the right to refuse treatment. Such is often the case for Jehovah's Witnesses, who refuse blood transfusions on religious grounds. In some situations, the court appoints a guardian who then may consent for the patient. This is especially true in the case of minors.

It is wise to check your state's Doctrine of Informed Consent for specific exceptions and information.

SPECIAL CONSENT TO OPERATION, POST OPERATIVE CARE,
MEDICAL TREATMENT, ANESTHESIA, OR OTHER PROCEDURE

Patient:_____ Patient No:_____

Washington State law guarantees that you have both the right and obligation to make decisions concerning your health care. Your physician can provide you with the necessary information and advice, but as a member of the health care team, you must enter into the decision making process. This form has been designed to acknowledge your acceptance of treatment recommended by your physician.

IMPORTANT: HAVE PATIENT SIGN FULL OR LIMITED DISCLOSURE BOX AND SIGNATURE LINE AT BOTTOM.

① I hereby authorize Dr._____
and/or such associates or assistants as may be selected by said physician to treat the following condition(s) which has (have) been explained to me: (Explain the nature of the condition(s) in professional and lay language.)

_____

_____

_____

Full Disclosure

I certify that my physician has informed me of the nature and character of the proposed treatment, of the anticipated results of the proposed treatment, of the possible alternative forms of treatment; and the recognized serious possible risks, complications, and the anticipated benefits involved in the proposed treatment and in the alternative forms of treatment, including non-treatment.

PATIENT/OTHER LEGALLY RESPONSIBLE PERSON SIGN
IF APPLICABLE

② The procedures planned for treatment of my condition(s) have been explained to me by my physician. I understand them to be: (Describe procedures to be performed in professional and lay language.)

_____

_____

_____

_____

Limited Disclosure

I certify that my physician has explained to me that I have the right to have clearly described to me the nature and character of the proposed treatment; the anticipated results of the proposed treatment; the alternative forms of treatment; and the recognized serious possible risks, complications, and anticipated benefits involved in the proposed treatment, and in the alternative forms of treatment, including non-treatment.

I do not wish to have these risks and facts explained to me.

At:_____
(NAME OF HOSPITAL OR MEDICAL FACILITY)

PATIENT/OTHER LEGALLY RESPONSIBLE PERSON SIGN
IF APPLICABLE

③ I recognize that, during the course of the operation, post operative care, medical treatment, anesthesia or other procedure, unforeseen conditions may necessitate additional or different procedures than those above set forth. **I therefore authorize my above named physician, and his or her assistants or designees, to perform such surgical or other procedures as are in the exercise of his, her or their professional judgment necessary and desirable.** The authority granted under this paragraph shall extend to the treatment of **all conditions** that require treatment and are not known to my physician at the time the medical or surgical procedure is commenced.

Any sections below which do not apply to the proposed treatment may be crossed out. All sections crossed out must be initialed by both physician and patient.

⑤ I consent to the administration of anesthesia by my attending physician, by an anesthesiologist, or other qualified party under the direction of a physician as may be deemed necessary. I understand that all anesthetics involve risks of complications and serious possible damage to vital organs such as the brain, heart, lung, liver and kidney and that in some cases may result in paralysis, cardiac arrest and/or brain death from both known and unknown causes.

④ **I have been informed that there are significant risks such as** severe loss of blood, infection and cardiac arrest that can lead to death or permanent or partial disability, which may be attendant to the performance of any procedure. I **acknowledge that no warranty or guarantee has been made to me as to result or cure.**

⑥ I consent to the use of transfusion of blood and blood products as deemed necessary.

⑦ Any tissues or parts surgically removed may be disposed of by the hospital or physician in accordance with accustomed practice.

I certify this form has been fully explained to me, that I have read it or have had it read to me, that the blank spaces have been filled in, and that I understand its contents.

DATE:_____ TIME:_____ A.M. P.M.

PATIENT/OTHER LEGALLY RESPONSIBLE PERSON SIGN

WITNESS:_____

RELATIONSHIP OF LEGALLY RESPONSIBLE PERSON TO PATIENT

FIGURE 9. Sample of Washington State informed consent form.

IMPLEMENTING CONSENT

Consent forms will be prepared for patients' signatures. The office staff may be responsible for the preparation of specifically designed forms or the procurement of preprinted consent forms (Figure 9). In either case, the form must be understandable, must protect the rights of the patient, must be broad enough to cover anything contemplated, but specific enough to make "informed consent." A so-called "blanket" consent form, which seeks to cover *all* aspects of patient care and is not specific, must be avoided.

Care should be given to be certain that all elements of informed consent have been understood by the patient before a signature is affixed. It is wise to include an expiration date to the consent. Another consideration may be allowing a waiting period between consent and administration of the procedure or treatment, the latter particularly in the case of sterilization.

You, as a medical office employee, may be asked to witness a signature that is a verification of the honest exchange between the physician and the patient. It is the physician who is responsible for the explanation of medical treatment to the patient, although you may provide reinforcement through clarification. If the patient has any further questions about the treatment or difficulties with the consent form, let the physician know. If the patient signs with an "X," two witnesses are required. It is advisable for the younger staff members to witness consent forms; this helps to assure the longevity of the witnesses should there be any problems in later years. There will be at least three copies of the signed consent form—one for the patient, one for the records, and one for the hospital, if necessary.

DISCUSSION QUESTIONS

1. Define:
   a. Consent
   b. Doctrine of Informed Consent.

2. Differentiate between informed and uninformed consent.

3. In an emergency situation, what type of consent exists? Explain and give an example.

4. The parents of a 6-year-old child consented to allow their daughter to undergo "routine cardiac tests." One of the tests performed was a catheter arteriogram where complications occurred. Questioning the parents revealed that they did not fully understand the risks involved. What are the legal implications of this consent? Identify potential problems in this situation.

5. What is the age of majority in your state?

6. A 15-year-old enters your office requesting treatment for scalds received on his hand while emptying the dishwasher at his place of employment. His family receives medical treatment at your office, but you are uncertain about seeing him without his parents' knowledge. Can he consent to treatment? What are the legal ramifications?

continues on next page

7. How specific should a consent form be? How general? Explain.

8. When you are asked to witness a signature, what does it legally mean?

9. An unmarried pregnant patient requests an abortion. Assuming the abortion is legal, what rights, if any, does the baby's father have in consent?

10. After a patient signed a consent form and you have witnessed it, she states, "I hope this is the right decision." What would you reply? What would you do?

CHAPTER 8

MEDICAL RECORDS

LEARNING OBJECTIVES

Upon successful completion of this chapter, you will:

1. Define medical records.

2. List six purposes of medical records in medical offices.

3. Name and define two types of charting.

4. Define SOAP and its use in medical records.

5. Demonstrate by example how and when to correct an error in medical records.

6. Define confidentiality and right to privacy as it relates to medical records.

7. Identify two circumstances in which a release of information is unnecessary.

8. Outline the process to follow when a subpoena is served.

9. Tell who owns medical records.

10. List and define two storage methods for medical records.

DEFINITIONS

Microform. Form used to produce microimages; that is, microfilm and microfiche.

Micrographics. Method of filing data on film using minute images.

POR or POMR. Problem-Oriented Records or Problem-Oriented Medical Records. A charting system developed by Lawrence L. Weed, M.D., that is based on patient problems.

SOAP. A charting method using Subjective and Objective data for patient Assessment and Planning.

INTRODUCTION

The development and care of medical records requires much attention of the medical office staff. Both employees and physicians will collect and enter data into patients' medical records. Medical records are a part of every person, beginning with the birth certificate and ending with the death certificate. With increased health awareness, patients are more concerned about what goes into their medical records. Patients also care who has access to their records. Are the records legal documents? Are they confidential? What authorization is required to release patients' medical records? Who owns them? These are questions medical office employees face daily.

The primary goal of any medical record is the proper care and identification of the patient. A patient's medical record that is accurate, complete, and concise encourages better medical care than a record that is not up-to-date and is a folder of loose papers not necessarily related or in order.

This chapter deals with medical records in physicians' offices rather than hospital medical records. While regulations for hospital records may be mandated by state statutes and requirements for hospital licensure, there are generally no such regulations for medical records in the office.

PURPOSES

The Joint Commission on Accreditation of Hospitals (JCAH) has established guidelines for medical records in the hospital.[1] Using these as a base, the primary purposes of medical records in the medical office are:

1. To provide a base for managing patient care, which includes initiating, diagnosing, implementing, and evaluating.
2. To provide inter- and intra-office communication of patient-related data.
3. To document total and complete health care from birth to death.
4. To allow patterns to surface that will alert physicians of patients' needs.
5. To serve as legal basis for evidence in litigation, and to protect legal interests of patients.
6. To provide clinical data for education and research.

The medical record is an official document of what has happened to the patient during a specific time. The type of charting and medical record used in medical offices varies. Specialists who see the patient only once may have an abbreviated form of medical record, merely a 5×8" card. By contrast, a physician who has had the same patient for thirty years may have three file folders with several hundred sheets of medical data on that patient. Whatever type is utilized, each patient needs a medical record.

POMR

One system of medical records is Problem-Oriented Medical Records (POMR) or Problem-Oriented Records (POR), a system developed by Dr. Lawrence L. Weed.[2] PORs are based on patients' problems, and every office employee, including the physician, charts in a particular place in the same manner. In source-oriented records, physicians chart in progress notes and nurses in nursing notes. PORs identify patient problems, not simply diagnoses, based on defined data. A problem can be a condition or a behavior that results in physical or emotional distress or interferes with the patient's functioning. Examples may include pain in knees and ankles, fear of falling, decreased appetite, and even inability to pay medical bills. The problem list is usually numbered, appears on the chart face sheet, and serves as a checklist to ascertain the patient's progress.

To identify patients' problems, the physician selects a data base that may include a physical examination, history, laboratory tests, and subjective data from the patient. Every problem has a plan and its progress is recorded in the medical record.

SOAP

The method of charting in PORs may vary widely; however, many offices use "SOAP"—subjective, objective, assessment, and plan. Once a problem is identified, it is "SOAPed."

Descriptions of SOAP are as follows:

S: Subjective: What subject or patient says; family comments, hearsay; patient's exact words are used.

O: Objective: Events that are directly observed or measurable; laboratory tests, x-ray results; physical examination findings.

A: Assessment: Physician's evaluation based on the subjective and objective data. S + O = A.

P: Plan: Treatment Plan; actions taken; may be further divided into (a) diagnostic, (b) therapeutic, and (c) educational.[3]

An example of the SOAP format is shown in Figure 10.

CALCANEO, Henry R.
08/18/40

Date of Onset	Date Recorded	PROBLEM LIST	Date Resolved	INACTIVE PROBLEMS
?	10/08/81	1. Increased appetite; increased thirst	10/20/81	
05/28/82	06/30/82	2. Dyspnea	07/10/82	
08/11/82	08/21/82	3. Loss of job		

10/08/81   1. Increased appetite, increased thirst

S: "I eat all the time & never gain wt. " " I didn't think about it, but yes, I drink all the time, too."

O: B/P 120/88. T—P—R: 98^9—80—18. Color good. Skin turger adequate. Wt. 5# less than 3 weeks ago. Urine, 4+ sugar. FBS, positive.

A: Uncontrolled diabetes; in family history.

P: Dx: Lab work-up for diabetes
    Tx: Begin on insulin, diabetic diet.
    Ed: Enroll in diabetic classes stat; instruct in diet and exercise.

06/30/82   2. Dyspnea

S: "I can't seem to get my breath. I'm weak all the time. It's worse when I lay down."

O: B/P 180/98. T—P—R: 99—88—26. Chest x-ray neg. Awakens from sleep with respiratory distress. Cough; slight edema.

A: Congestive heart failure, left sided. History of hypertension & diabetes.

P: Hospitalize for cardiac workup.

08/21/82   3. Loss of Job

S: "What can I do now? I'm not trained for anything but construction, & with this heart problem, I'll never get back my old job."

O: Heart condition improved; wt. gain 30#; brittle diabetic.

A: Doesn't seem worried about A JOB; is upset that current job is not available to him now. Off diet.

P: Send to rehab for evaluation & training for new profession; stress diet & exercise; lose 20 lbs.

FIGURE 10. Sample of SOAP in chart.

SOAP also may be found in a source-oriented medical record, which is more likely a collection of narrative pages. Each time the patient is seen by the physician, an entry is made, handwritten by the physician or dictated and then typed by an employee. Laboratory and x-ray results are collected together, may be color coded, and may be shingled or layered in chronological order.

Whatever method of charting is utilized in medical records, it is important to be concise, complete, clear, and chronological.

USE OF RECORDS IN LITIGATION

If an error is made on a medical record, it must be properly corrected. Errors made while typing should be corrected as any other typewritten material would be. Handwritten errors and typed errors discovered later should be corrected by the following method: Draw a line through the error, write "correction" or "corr.," sign your initials, indicate the date, and write in the correction. When erasures or obliterations occur, confusion and suspicion may result.

What is in the medical record is confidential. Any employees handling records must protect the privacy of patients unless otherwise required by law. Some states will consider the communication between patient and physician to be privileged. The privilege belongs to patients and is important because physicians will need to know very personal and private information about patients during the course of their treatment.

No information should be released from the medical record without the physician's approval and written permission of the patient—and then only the specific information authorized should be released. It may be helpful for the medical office to create a form that may be signed by patients for the release of any medical records. The simplest release is seen on many insurance claim forms, which require the patient's signature before certain data are released to the insurance carrier.

If the patient is a minor or is incompetent, the legal guardian may sign the release of information. If the patient is deceased, the personal representative of the estate is allowed to sign.[4] Recent laws have allowed some government and state agencies, such as those that administer the Medicaid program, access to medical records without patients' consent. A standard procedure to follow is essential for maintaining confidentiality and good patient relations.

There are times during the course of medical practice when a patient's chart will be subpoenaed by a court of law. It is advisable to notify the patient when releasing the record in accordance with the subpoena. Unless the original is subpoenaed, a certified, photostatic copy should be made for the courts. If the original is subpoenaed, a copy should be made to remain in the office. An original medical record is best hand-delivered to the clerk of the court and a receipt obtained. The cost of making copies is usually paid by the person or agency issuing the subpoena.

Physicians and employees also will want to remember that the medical record may be as valuable for what it does not say as for what it does say. An act not recorded is generally considered an act not done by most courts of law. The necessity for using a medical record in a court emphasizes the importance of accurate records that honestly reflect the patient's course of treatment. A record that is readable, understandable, and complete will better withstand the scrutiny in a courtroom.

OWNERSHIP OF MEDICAL RECORDS

The accepted rule is that medical records are the property of the person(s) entering the data in them. Physicians are considered the owners of the medical records they have written.

In recent years, patients increasingly have been allowed access to their medical records. Some state medical societies encourage the release of a copy of the medical record to a patient. Patients can be expected to make an appointment and pay reproduction fees. When patients have been denied access to their records, attorneys have been employed to obtain copies of the records. Access should be withheld only when the law prohibits such access, or when, in the physician's opinion, great harm would be done to the patient.

Patients who request that their medical records be transferred to another physician should do so in writing. The original record may be retained in the office and the request honored with a photostatic copy of the complete record or the physician's summary. The continuance of medical records is quite important in a society that is so mobile. This continuity can be accomplished only with cooperation from physicians. A small fee may be charged for copying the record. The important factor is to release the record promptly so that the patient can receive proper care from the new physician.

Medical office employees must be especially cautious with automated medical records. The increased use of computers and word processing equipment in medical offices for both financial and health records makes confidential information fairly accessible. The storage of health data and information has valuable possibilities for improving health care, but also may lead to an unnecessary invasion of patients' privacy.

RETENTION OF MEDICAL RECORDS

How long to retain medical records is not easily established. One guideline indicates that records should be retained until the statute of limitations for acts of medical malpractice has run out so records are available for any possible litigation. This guideline may require a pediatrician to keep the record for as long as six years beyond the age of majority.

It is probably wise for physicians to keep medical records of patients permanently. In the future, family medical records may be as important as the individual medical record. It may be valuable for children to have their deceased parents' medical histories added to their own. Recent medical developments show that medications taken by mothers during pregnancy may affect their children in later years. Much patient care for illnesses is directly related to genetic makeup. Without family records, full disclosure and study may be impaired.

These suggestions will cause employees and their physicians to cringe when thinking of the warehouse they may have to rent to store all the data collected during the course of their patients' treatment.

STORAGE OF MEDICAL RECORDS

Not all medical records need to be kept in the same location. The "active" records should be in readiness for physicians. The "closed" files usually include records of patients who are no longer being seen by the physician, who may have moved away, or who have died. These files may be kept in a storage area separate from the current and active files. The office may have basement space or physicians may even rent storage space in another location.

MICROGRAPHICS

If storage space is at a premium, micrographics may provide a solution. Micrographics is a method of filing data on film using minute (micro) images. There are two common microforms often used in the medical office: (1) microfilm, and (2) microfiche.[5]

Microfilm prints the pertinent information from the medical record on a roll film. A 100-foot roll of 16 mm film is stored in containers about $4 \times 4 \times 1''$. The material contained in this size container is roughly equivalent to one file drawer of medical records. A piece of equipment, a reader, is necessary for viewing the information after it has been microfilmed.[6]

Microfiche is a small sheet of microfilm about $4 \times 6''$ that contains information to be stored. The process is much the same except that the material is on sheets rather than film rolls. Microfiche storage requires less space than does microfilm. Again, additional equipment is necessary to view the information.

Before storing data on any microform, a cost comparison should be done, considering the process and equipment to purchase or rent as well as the space saved. Other considerations are (1) how long the record is to be kept, (2) how frequently retrieval will be necessary, and (3) the importance of any color coding, which is very difficult to reproduce on regular microforms.

Much personnel time is required to prepare files for filming. Time must be spent:

1. Removing any staples or fasteners.
2. Arranging records in a predetermined sequence.
3. Removing any unnecessary papers.

4. Checking names and numbers for accuracy.
5. Making a divider sheet to separate individual records.[7]

These tasks are difficult to complete in regular working hours where there are many interruptions. It may be wise to hire outside assistance for the task or to pay office employees for additional hours.

There are professional firms whose business is the conversion of records to a microform for storage. They are able to advise and establish a system appropriate for any particular needs.

All persons involved in health care need to know how to manage medical records legally, including record creation, storage, retrieval, releasing, and disposal. Written office procedures for medical records need to be strictly followed. Handling medical records tends to be tedious and time-consuming, but without proper records patient care would be very difficult. Medical records are a vital part of the medical office and employees responsible for their care and upkeep should take pride in the knowledge that their work will be displayed in the medical record for many years to come.

REFERENCES

1.   HUFFMAN, EK: *Medical Records Management.* Physicians' Record Company, Berwyn, Illinois, 1978, p 33.

2.   WEED, LL: *Implementing the Problem-Oriented Medical Record,* ed 2. MCSA, Seattle, Washington, 1976.

3.   BERNI, R AND READEY, H: *Problem Oriented Medical Record Implementation.* CV Mosby, St Louis, 1974, p 54.

4.   *Patient Information Guide for Health Care Providers in Washington State.* Washington State Medical Record Association, 1979, pp 1-4.

5.   BERGERUD, M AND GONGOLY, J: *Word/Information Processing Concepts.* John Wiley and Sons, New York, 1981, p 138.

6.   HUFFMAN, p 231.

7.   IBID, p 236.

DISCUSSION QUESTIONS

1. Compare source-oriented and problem-oriented medical records.

2. While you are preparing the patient for the physician, the patient picks up the medical record and begins to read it. What do you do?

3. The following report was phoned in and charted.
"Urinalysis 08/16/82 reveals RBC too numerous to count."
When the written report was received, you note it is WBC, not RBC. Properly correct.

4. You are preparing a medical record after it has been subpoenaed. Describe the procedures you would follow.

5. A patient becomes angry when refused permission to hand-carry medical records when moving out of state. What alternatives can an employee suggest?

6. Describe what might be done when there is simply no room for any more medical records in the office.

CHAPTER 9

COLLECTION PRACTICES

LEARNING OBJECTIVES

Upon successful completion of this chapter, you will:

1. Explain, in a short paragraph, the importance of collections.

2. List three elements established by the Medical Group Management Association for collections.

3. List at least five appropriate items to be covered in a collection policy.

4. Identify the seven appropriate procedures to follow when collecting a bill by telephone or by mail.

5. Identify seven *Collection Don'ts* established by the Federal Trade Commission.

6. Explain the one important procedure to follow if a patient is denied credit because of a poor credit rating.

7. List nine steps to follow in selecting a collection agency.

8. Write a brief paragraph describing how personal feelings about individuals' ability to pay may influence their care.

INTRODUCTION

The collection of accounts belongs mostly to the business aspect of the medical office. Physicians may feel it is not appropriate for them to discuss financial matters with their patients, and prefer not to be involved with the day-to-day task of collections. Medical office employees generally avoid the task as long as possible, feeling that collections do not deserve the same level of importance as does direct patient care.

It is important to remember, however, that patients may become dissatisfied over collection of a fee more readily than over negligence. A reason for this may be that patients often protect their money more than their personal well-being. Many patients have been angered over an incorrect statement, a change to computer billing that prints overdue notices, or a situation when a medical office employee cannot answer financial questions over the telephone.

It is true that physicians are expected to treat the person rather than to collect the bill, and may not have time to devote to the financial practices of the office. Yet every office employee knows how important the total of the month's receipts is to the physician. Medical office employees who feel this task has less importance than direct patient care should remember that financial dealings with the patient allow them to care for the "whole" person. Many lawsuits have their inception in the front office over financial matters. Therefore, it is appropriate to discuss collections.

For the most part, the days of physicians rendering their services in exchange for a dozen eggs or wood for their stoves are gone. Physicians have a right to be reimbursed for the services they perform. It has taken many years of training and education to allow them to practice medicine. Their office equipment and supplies are costly. There should be no hesitancy by physicians or their employees to charge adequate fees for services rendered.

TRUTH IN LENDING ACT

Regulation Z of the Consumer Protection Act of 1968 also is known as the Truth in Lending Act. This Act is enforced by the Federal Trade Commission and when applied to medical offices deals with collection of patients' payments.

Briefly, the regulation requires that an agreement by physicians and their patients for payment of their medical bills in more than four installments *must* be in writing and must provide information regarding finance charges. Even if no finance charge is involved, the agreement must be in writing and stipulate no finance charge.

If patients decide to pay their bills by installments unilaterally with no established agreement with physicians, Regulation Z is not applicable so long as the physician's office continues to bill for the full amount.

Situations where the Truth in Lending Act is often used include arrangements for surgery, orthodontia, and prenatal and/or delivery care. The amount owed by the patient is often more than a patient can pay in one installment or is more than is covered by medical insurance. Office employees then can discuss with the patients appropriate installment payments, put the agreement in writing, and provide a copy for the patient. Few physicians will charge a finance fee in this situation, although to do so is both legal and ethical. If bilateral installment agreements are fairly common in your medical office or if computer billing automatically includes a finance charge after a certain period of time, it is wise to have the wording approved by an official of the Federal Trade Commission.

COLLECTION GUIDELINES

The Medical Group Management Association suggests three elements for collections that are worth noting. They are: (1) Collections must provide enough money to maintain the clinic and satisfy the physicians; (2) collection procedures must be firm enough to be effective; (3) collections must be temperate enough not to irritate otherwise satisfied patients who intend to pay.

How to establish fees is not discussed, but if the physicians' fees are consistent with those charged by others in the same community who perform similar tasks, there should be no difficulty with patients feeling that their bills are unreasonable. There should be no hesitancy on the part of physicians to discuss directly with patients the fees for their services. Many times, a patient will more readily accept a statement of fees from a doctor than from an office assistant.

Medical offices must establish an appropriate collection policy for employees to follow. That policy should determine if and at what point collection letters will be sent. Will they be on printed forms or personal letters? Will there be a minimum payment schedule? Will it be different for every patient? Are collection telephone calls to be made? If so, by whom? How many? When? What procedures will be followed? Will delinquent accounts ever be turned over to a collection agency or pursued through the local courts? A clearly defined or stated policy allows employees the support necessary to provide the firmness needed for collections to be successful.

COLLECTION DO'S

The following guidelines are provided to suggest possible procedures for collections in the medical office:

1. Establish appropriate fees for the services rendered in accordance with community guidelines and practices.
2. Discuss fees with patients the first time they present themselves at the office or call for treatment. A written payment and/or collection statement may prove useful.

3. Expect first-time patients to pay cash at the end of their visits.

4. Provide patients with an office brochure that gives them information about hours, emergency contacts, physicians' services, how billing is handled, and whom to call if there is a question about a bill. The brochure also should describe how insurance is handled.

5. Provide an opportunity for the patient to pay before leaving the office. The "super bill" is an ideal way for the physician to circle charges and services rendered as well as the diagnoses. The bill then is presented to patients and they are asked to stop at the receptionist's desk on their way out. The receptionist should never say, "Shall we bill you?" The receptionist should say, "Mrs. Lotta M. Bucks, your charge today is $35.00. Would you like to pay by cash or check?" Some offices have been very successful in providing patients with a stamped, addressed envelope to mail in the fee when they return home. Other offices do their first billing when the patient is ready to leave rather than at the end of the month.

6. If your office uses computer billing, explain the process to patients. Notify them when you move to a computer system so they will understand the changes and any problems that may occur.

7. Have an established practice for mailing out your statements and follow that practice. Statements should be itemized, accurate, and easy to understand. They should be mailed to arrive the first of the month. Statements that include envelopes are paid faster.

8. When your collection policy dictates that a bill should be followed with a letter or a telephone call, do it. Be consistent, pleasant, and firm. The sooner you follow up on a delinquent account, the more likely it will be collected.

9. Employees responsible for collections should have certain phrases and the wording of possible letters at their fingertips for quick and easy referral. They also need the authority to carry the collection process to its completion.

10. Suggested procedures for mail or telephone follow-up include:
    A. Introduction or greeting.
    B. Establish that you are speaking to the proper person, if it is a telephone call, or address a letter to the proper person.
    C. State the reason for the call or the letter. ("Your account is past due.")
    D. Be pleasant, but firm. ("You are generally prompt with your payments; we wondered if this has been overlooked.")
    E. Get a commitment. Make it specific. ("May we expect $35 from you by next Monday?") Then mark that commitment in your tickler file and follow-up next Monday if there has been no response.

      F. End the contact graciously. Do not get "pulled into" all the financial problems of the patient.

      G. Be prepared to offer a payment plan that is suitable both to the patient and to the physician.

11. Have a clearly established practice of when to turn the account over to a collection agency, to collect the balance due in small claims court, or to write off the balance as a loss.

COLLECTION DON'TS

The Federal Trade Commission has specific regulations for debt collection. They include:

1. Do not misrepresent who you are or why you are contacting a person.
2. Do not send "blind" post cards or notices saying "Please call me," signed "Janet."
3. Do not use deception in any form in your contact.
4. Do not telephone at odd hours, make repeated calls, calls to debtor's friends, relatives, neighbors, employers, or children. Acceptable hours to call are 8 A.M. to 8 P.M.
5. Do not threaten or falsely assert that credit ratings will be hurt.
6. Do not make calls or send letters demanding payment for amounts not owed.
7. If a contact must be made to the debtor's place of business, do not reveal to a third party the reason for the contact. The patient's privacy and reputation must be protected.

If your office denies credit to a patient on the basis of an adverse credit report from a credit bureau or similar agency, *you must volunteer* the name and address of the agency providing the information to the patient, even if you are not asked. Failure to do so could result in legal action. It may be wise to have a form letter available in your office that courteously informs the patient that credit has been denied, leaving blanks for the name and address of the agency which supplied the credit information. Mail a copy to the patient and keep a copy for your records.

COLLECTION PROBLEMS

The "up-front, matter-of-fact" approach to collections will increase the cash flow in the medical office and make collections easier for everyone. However, every office has slow payers, hardship cases, and deadbeats. Try to move slow payers to a cash basis as soon and as often as possible and yet maintain good public relations.

Hardship cases pose another problem. Any of us could reach a time in our lives when the payment of a medical bill might be nearly impossible. Care must be taken to be understanding at all times. Try to work out minimal payment plans with the patients so that they, too, are able to sense pride in themselves and their ability to pay. Social agencies may be suggested if necessary. If circumstances dictate, physicians may choose to write off an account rather than try to collect. That is a decision for the physician.

The deadbeat is still another problem. There will always be a small percentage of patients who never intend to pay their bills. All possible resources should be exhausted in a courteous manner, but the accounts then should be taken to small claims court or turned over to a collection agency. It is fairly common for physicians to withdraw themselves formally from these cases and encourage the patients to seek treatment elsewhere.

Chapter 1 gives information about the procedures to follow for collecting a bill from the estate of a patient who has died. Also in Chapter 1 is an explanation of the steps to follow for taking a patient to small claims court. Both of the situations are fairly uncomplicated and will warrant results worth the effort if employees are consistent and conscientious in these dealings.

COLLECTION AGENCIES

If you have diligently followed your billing and collection procedures and come to the conclusion that the patient is not going to pay, you have two options. One option is to write off the account; the other is to turn it over to a collection agency. Obviously, this decision must be consistent with office policy while still vesting the final decision in the physician.

Collection agencies are generally employed as a last resort. Most people, including patients and physicians, tend to have a negative attitude toward collection agencies. However, the agency can be valuable to physicians who choose to utilize such professional services.

Selection of an appropriate agency should be made as carefully as one would choose a bank. Investigation includes:

1) Does it handle medical-dental accounts exclusively?
2) What methods does it use to collect?
3) What is the agency's financial responsibility?
4) What percentage will the medical office receive?
5) How promptly does it settle accounts?
6) Does the agency have a good bank reference?
7) How much cost versus goodwill will your office incur by using this agency?
8) Will it provide you with a list of satisfied customers or references?
9) Will you have the ability to end the agency's collection efforts?

It is a good idea to check with the Better Business Bureau or the local medical society for possible recommendations. If the agency is a member of the American Collectors Association, it will generally adhere to high ethical standards.

Once the agency is selected, all the delinquent accounts need to be turned over to it, including any useful nonclinical data. The medical office should keep a record of what has been given to the agency as well as a running account of the agency's progress. Any contact, whether it be in person, via phone, or via letter, should cease once the account has been turned over to the collection agency. If the patient sends payment to the office, report it immediately to the agency. If patients call, courteously refer them to the agency.

The collection agency is representing the physician and medical office. Office employees should work with the agency to collect the accounts. Success by an agency nearly all the time in collecting accounts may be indicative of a medical office staff that lacks sufficient training to be effective in collections.

COLLECTIONS AND ATTITUDES

The patients' financial status has no bearing on the kind of treatment they should receive in the medical office. The Medicaid patient should receive the same care as the patient who pays cash. Physicians and employees need to be careful of their attitudes toward those patients who have difficulty paying their bill, for whatever reason. Actions often speak louder than words, and patients easily perceive their true meanings.

RESOURCES

Valuable seminars are frequently presented by medical societies or private consulting firms that can assist medical employees in the collection of accounts. Such seminars are a wise investment for physicians. The Medical Group Management Association publishes a book, *Medical Credit and Collections*, which also is helpful. It can be obtained by writing to its offices at 4101 East Louisiana Avenue, Denver, CO 80222. The American Medical Association's booklet *The Business Side of Medical Practice* has a suggested "Collection Timetable" and an "Aids and Checklist," which also is beneficial. It is available through AMA at P.O. Box 821, Monroe, WI 53566.

DISCUSSION QUESTIONS

1. As a newly employed medical office manager, you discover that one of the physicians in the office does not follow the written
continues on next page

collections policies and is more lenient about patients paying their bills. What problem does this create for you and the other physicians?

2. A physician overhears the receptionist say to a patient, "Well, you know, we can take only so many welfare patients." How can the patient now be put at ease?

3. The office has just converted to computer billing. A patient encloses a note with a check that says, "Now I guess I'm just a number in your office, too. I don't like your new bills." What course of action would you suggest?

4. Correct the following telephone conversation:

Bookkeeper (BK): "Hi, this is Dr. Erythro's office. Who's this?"

Patient (PT): "This is Laura Phagocyte."

BK: "You owe us $46.20. Can you pay us $10 today?"

PT: "Yeah. I'll put it in the mail."

BK: "Will it be check or money order?"

PT: "Check."

BK: "Fine, I'll expect it in a few days. Thank you. Goodbye."

CHAPTER 10

HIRING PRACTICES

LEARNING OBJECTIVES

Upon successful completion of this chapter, you will:

1. Explain, in your own words, the importance of correct hiring practices.

2. Recall one source of information on hiring practices beneficial to physicians.

3. List at least four necessary components of personnel policies.

4. Identify the three necessary elements of job descriptions.

5. Discuss office hours, work week, benefits, and salaries.

6. Explain, in your own words, where and how to locate prospective employees.

7. List eight techniques to effective interviews.

8. Identify the five potential discrimination problems to consider when hiring.

9. Recall procedures for selecting the right employee.

10. Recognize steps that encourage employee longevity.

INTRODUCTION

Few physicians function alone in the medical office. Even physicians first setting up practice as sole proprietors will hire an assistant as soon as possible. Selecting appropriate personnel is an important business task. Frequently, office employees will be influential and/or directly involved in the process of hiring additional employees. Hiring and preparing employees to function in specific roles is both expensive and time consuming. Some major areas of consideration are:

1. Personnel policies
2. Job descriptions
3. Employee evaluations
4. Locating employees
5. Interview process
6. Selecting employees
7. Keeping employees.

Valuable information is found in *The Business Side of Medical Practice,* published by the American Medical Association. The chapter "As Your Practice Grows" provides an excellent discussion of hiring practices for the medical office.

PERSONNEL POLICIES

Without established personnel policies, physicians soon lose control of the management of their own practice. Before the first person is hired, physicians must determine their office needs, job descriptions, office hours and work week, benefits and salaries, and how employees will be evaluated. Physicians will need to determine if their employees are to be generalists or specialists in their skills, or if a combination of employees would be more effective.

Once these personnel policies have been determined, they should be set down in writing in an office procedural manual. The policies should be updated from time to time to reflect any changes in the office, but they should always be in writing and available to employees. Once personnel policies have been established, prospective employees' questions can be answered.

JOB DESCRIPTIONS

Job descriptions indicate minimum qualifications, a description of the jobs to be performed, and to whom the employee is responsible. Written job descriptions are often shared with candidates at the time of interviews.

When a new office is opened, job descriptions will have to be developed. *The Business Side of Medical Practice,* mentioned earlier, gives samples for study. Other medical offices and/or office managers may be willing to share job descriptions used in their office. Medical assistant educators and professional organizations also are a helpful resource.

The established medical office will find its employees to be the best resources when writing job descriptions. Job descriptions are established by having the employees put in writing descriptions of the tasks they perform in a normal work day. This exercise provides the base for the job descriptions.

OFFICE HOURS AND WORK WEEK

Office hours and the work week are generally easier to establish than job descriptions. Hours may be determined by the medical specialty as well as the dictates of the community. It is important to provide for the long and often inconsistent hours of a medical practice. For example, will every employee stay late, will hours be staggered, will overtime be compensated? Will the work week be the same or longer than office hours? How will a policy be established that provides for the needs of patients and allows all tasks to be performed?

Many employees become unhappy when they are told in the beginning that the work week will be 40 hours, and it turns out the work week is closer to 50 or 60 hours. Planning for overtime is essential.

BENEFITS AND SALARIES

Benefits and salaries are of concern both to employees and employers. Physicians should pay a salary that first is commensurate with the responsibilities of the task to be performed and second, that takes into consideration education, training, and experience of the employees. A third consideration can be the prevailing wage of the community.

Benefits to consider include medical, sick leave, vacations, holidays, retirement, and profit-sharing plans. Other incentives may include payment of educational courses and seminars, and uniform allowance. An important benefit, especially in the city, may be free parking.

EMPLOYEE EVALUATIONS

Evaluation of employees is an ongoing task throughout the individual's employment. Seldom, however, it is a formal process. Yet this probably is the biggest mistake made in employment. A clearly established and written evaluation policy and form should be determined. It should be carefully explained to employees and a copy should be available to them. At regular intervals during the course of employment, managers should discuss the evaluation with their employees. Areas of strengths as well as weaknesses should be documented. The evaluation then should become part of the employees' personnel file.

An adequate evaluation enables employees to improve job performances, serves as a tool for employers to discuss salary increases, provides background for any necessary dismissal, and establishes a record for future referral. Note the sample patterned after a "Review of Progress" from *The Business Side of Medical Practice* (Figure 11).

LOCATING EMPLOYEES

A valuable resource for medical offices seeking employees is the county medical society. Some medical societies may sponsor a medical employment agency. Schools in the community that have accredited training programs for medical assistants and medical secretaries often have names of graduates seeking employment.

Professional organizations such as the American Association of Medical Assistants (a national organization for medical office assistants that may have a local chapter in your community) may be able to provide possible candidates for employment.

Other physicians and their employees often know of potential candidates. Employment agencies specializing in medical and dental employment are other sources. Newspaper advertising may be successful.

In an established medical practice, the initial screening of candidates often is delegated to an office manager or a specific person other than the physician.

INTERVIEW PROCESS

With a printed job description and a list of possible candidates, the interview process can begin. The interview is a time to meet with each candidate personally. A job application may or may not have been completed at this point.

McDouble[1] in "A Memo to Interviewers" cites some common-sense techniques to make the interview more effective.

1. Identify the purpose of the interview and follow through with it.
2. Avoid interruptions during the interview. Don't rush.
3. Utilize effective communication skills and listen carefully to the candidate.
4. Observe nonverbal behavior.
5. Ask each candidate the same questions. These may include:
   a. What are your qualifications?
   b. Why are you leaving your present position?
   c. When can you begin work?
   d. What salary do you expect?
   e. What do you expect to be doing in one year? In five years?
   f. Why do you want to work here?

PROGRESS REVIEW

Name _____

Position _____

Date Hired _____

Starting Salary _____

Job Knowledge	Thoroughly understands all aspects.	More than adequate knowledge of job.	Has sufficient knowledge to do job.	Insufficient knowledge of some phases.	Continually needs instruction/supervision.

Comments: _____

Quality of Work	Always neat, Accurate and thorough.	Only a few mistakes— careful worker.	Work is acceptable.	Occasionally careless—needs checking.	Inaccurate and careless.

Comments: _____

Cooperation	Exceptional team worker: flexible.	Usually agreeable. Tactful and obliging.	Goes along satisfactorily.	Sometimes difficult to work with.	Works poorly with others.

Comments: _____

Responsibility	Accepts all responsibilities fully; meets emergencies.	Conscientiously tries to fulfill job responsibilities.	Accepts but does not seek responsibility.	Does some assigned tasks reluctantly.	Often indifferent; avoids responsibilities.

Comments: _____

continues on next page

FIGURE 11. Sample of employee evaluation form. Adapted from *The Business Side of Medical Practice*, American Medical Association, Monroe, Wisconsin, 1979, pp. 73–74.

Initiative	Self-starter: makes practical suggestions.	Proceeds on assigned work voluntarily and readily accepts suggestions.	Does regular work without prompting.	Relies on others; needs help getting started.	Must usually be told exactly what to do.
Comments:				
Quantity of Work	Maintains high output.	Usually does more than expected.	Does required work.	Inclined to be slow.	Others may need to help complete work.
Comments:				
Dependability	Places company interests ahead of personal conveniences.	Punctual—does not waste time.	Generally on the job as needed.	Some abuses— occasionally needs to be admonished.	Abuses work schedule often.
Comments:				
Leadership/ Supervision	Exceptional leader and organizer.	Poised and is respected by other workers.	Has adequate leadership qualities.	Shy; needs leadership development.	Not an organizer. Does not inspire others.
Comments:				

In What Ways Has This Individual Definitely Grown? _____

What Are the Strong Points? _____

In What Way Has the Individual Failed to Grow? _____

What Are the Weak Points? _____

Days Absent This Period _____

Office Time (Paid) _____

Own Time (Non-Paid) _____

Number Sick Days _____

This Review for the Period _____ to _____ 19 _____

Would You Recommend Rehire _____ (Yes)
_____ (No)

Complete if Employee Is Leaving The Office: _____

Why? _____

Reviewing Physician/Administrator: _____

Discussed with Employee on: _____
(Date)

g. Do you foresee any difficulties that may prevent you from doing a good job?
6. Remain objective.
7. Maintain control of the interview.
8. End on a positive note; summarize; provide candidate with a possible date for a decision.

Following each interview, take the time to make any notes that will serve as a reminder later when considering several candidates.

LEGAL IMPLICATIONS

Individuals involved in the hiring process need to be knowledgeable of their state and Federal work and employment regulations. The Department of Labor, Wage and Hour Division, will answer questions regarding minimum wages, use of child labor, and length of work. Your state Human Rights Commission will be able to answer questions on possible discrimination in the interview and/or hiring process.

The Federal law states that an employer of fifteen or more must not discriminate on any form of application for employment, or during any inquiry in connection with prospective employment. The discrimination includes age, sex, race, creed, marital status, national origin, color or handicaps (sensory, mental, or physical). State laws may be more strict than Federal law. For example, in Washington an employer of eight or more cannot discriminate.

Nothing in either the Federal or state discrimination laws is intended to prevent the employer from hiring only qualified persons. Obviously, to protect this right, a well-written job description is essential.

Potential discrimination problem areas include:

1. *Age:* Any inquiry that implies a preference is prohibited. Age and birthdate may be requested.
2. *Marital Status:* No inquiries permitted.
3. *Race or Color:* No inquiry concerning race or color of skin, hair, eyes, and so forth is permitted.
4. *Sex:* No inquiry permitted.
5. *Handicap:* No inquiry if handicaps or health problems are not related to job performance. If employer should take handicap into account in determining job placement or fitness to perform, then inquiry can be made.

Most laws permit employers to talk about the job, its duties, and responsibilities, but prohibit any questions unrelated to the job. For example, it is *not* job-related to note that the applicant has children, but it *is* job-related to note whether the applicant indicated problems getting to work or working overtime.

It is important to prepare for the interview by bringing a structured outline of subjects to cover with all applicants. Treat them alike in all respects whether they are male or female.

Some valid reasons for declining applicants may include:

1. Applicant has health problem that would preclude the safe and efficient performance of the job.
2. Applicant is not fully available for the work schedule of the particular job (religion observance not included).
3. Insufficient skills training or experience to perform the duties of the particular job.
4. Another applicant is better qualified.[2]

Even though the medical office may not have fifteen, or even eight employees, it is wise to follow the state and federal requirements, not only for protection but also for ethical reasons, and good public relations.

SELECTING EMPLOYEES

After completion of the interview process, it is advisable to make a careful study of all the candidates and their responses to questions. Employment applications should be read, and references should be contacted. Talking with former employers and individuals named as references is a most important part of the decision-making process.

How each candidate will function with other staff members should be considered. If candidates have been asked to perform any skill functions, they should be checked for accuracy. Candidates may be asked to do some typewriting, take a spelling test (medical and nonmedical words), or perform a clinical function. It is wise to phone candidates themselves or ask them to phone the office at a later time to screen their telephone personalities. The manner in which candidates handle the telephone is important, since the patient's first contact with the doctor is often over the telephone.

Once a decision is made, all candidates should be informed. This is a courtesy often overlooked. It may be wise to establish a probationary period for the new employee. A period of three months is usually adequate time to determine if the working relationship is a good one. At the end of this period, either employee or employer should feel free to terminate if there is any reason to feel the agreement is not a lasting one. Salary paid during the probationary period may be less than is offered at the end of that time.

KEEPING EMPLOYEES

Keeping employees is as important as selecting them. Salaries that are commensurate with work performance and the qualifications of employees are a must. Salary is not a place to try to cut office expense. The old adage "You get what you pay for" is true in employment.

As important to employees as an adequate salary is the assurance that their work is appreciated and is necessary for efficient functioning in the medical office. "Thank you" and "Well done" are compliments that foster goodwill and motivate employees to greater effectiveness. Good employees merit your trust and increased responsibilities. Encourage employees to improve their education and knowledge, and provide incentives for that. If employees are to be corrected or disciplined, never do so in front of other employees or patients. Most will accept criticism well if it is done tactfully. Few will forget if they are embarrassed before their peers or the patients. Remembering birthdays and the anniversaries of employment with simple gifts or cards takes little effort, but does much for employee morale.

Employees in the office can make or break a successful medical practice. It is important to take the time and effort to insure that the office staff functions as a "team" to create an atmosphere conducive to good physician-patient relationships.

REFERENCES

1. McDouble, LG: *A memo to interviewers.* Supervisory Management, New York, May 1978, pp 118-119.
2. Fullner, W: *Complying with the State Law Against Discrimination in Employment.* Association of Washington Business in cooperation with the Washington State Human Rights Commission.

DISCUSSION QUESTIONS

1. In seeking a medical office employee, describe three places where you might look and give the reasons for your selection.

2. When interviewing a candidate, a question is asked that the candidate refuses to answer, citing discrimination as a reason. What should you do?

3. How could the following situation be prevented by using wise employment practices?
    The physician is speaking to the assistant in the hall.
    "I'm tired of telling you how to do things and having you mess it up during an exam. Pick up your check at the end of the week and don't come back."

4. Under what conditions might office hours and employee work week be different. Why?

5. Dream a little. You have the "perfect" employee and want to show your appreciation. What might you do?

6. Conduct an interview for employment.

CHAPTER 11

INTRODUCTION TO ETHICS AND BIOETHICS

LEARNING OBJECTIVES

Upon successful completion of this chapter, you will

1. Define ethics and bioethics.
2. Explain why ethics and bioethics are necessary in the practice of medicine.
3. List and discuss at least five ethical codes.
4. Recall some bioethical issues in medicine.

INTRODUCTION

Nearly everyone has experienced the sensation of "feeling less than human" in the physician's office. It tends to be dehumanizing to be stripped of your clothing and placed prone on an uncomfortable table, then expected to answer the questions of the physician or respond to the medical office employee. Such situations are basic reasons for ethical standards.

Ethics are not easy to define, but they generally relate to what is right or wrong and to a set of moral values. Ethics also refer to the various codes of conduct that have been established through the years by members of the medical profession. But it is not appropriate today to consider ethical standards without a discussion of bioethics. Bioethics refer to the moral issues and problems that have arisen as a result of today's modern medicine and research. Both ethics and bioethics will be discussed.

WHY ARE MEDICAL ETHICS IMPORTANT?

A reasonable question is: "Why are medical ethics necessary?" To offer an adequate answer, one must consider the climate of the medical office today.

Why is it that many medical offices have more patients than they can adequately treat? Why do many patients feel their physician does not care for them as a "whole person?" Why are patients more involved in their medical care now than fifty years ago? Questions such as these reflect the medical climate in today's offices.

To attempt to understand this climate, consider how expensive it is to go to medical school today. Unless a student has independent wealth, it is very likely that aspiring new physicians have a heavy indebtedness to overcome as soon as they begin to practice. A patient load that is too heavy for one physician to handle adequately may result.

Medical students work hard, long hours during their training and internship, often for very little remuneration. They learn early that they must be objective about patients to survive the mental strain. Such a need may foster an attitude that eliminates concern for anything but the patient's disorder. Another factor to consider is that the advances in medical research (none of which we would like to forfeit) demand a heavy science background for physicians. The opportunity for learning how to relate and communicate well with patients may be far down on the list of curriculum requirements.[1]

Patients are much more knowledgeable today about their health. Therefore, patients are apt to demand more from physicians, may question the validity of tests, and are more likely to speak out against the high cost of medical care.

All of these factors have an influence on physicians and medical office employees. Knowledge of ethical codes and a sympathetic understanding of bioethical issues will enable physicians, medical office employees, and patients to work together for better medical care.

Complete transcripts of the various ethical codes to be considered can be found at the end of this chapter, but a brief summary of each follows.

The Hippocratic Oath, while not as prominent in medical schools today, still may be found on the walls of many medical offices and clinics. It was first written in the fifth century B.C. It was later Christianized in the tenth or eleventh century A.D. to eliminate referral to pagan gods. The Hippocratic Oath protected the rights of patients and appealed to the inner and finer instincts of the physician *without* imposing penalties.

The Geneva Convention Code of Medical Ethics established by the World Medical Association in 1949 is similar to the Hippocratic Oath. This code refers to "colleagues as brothers" and states that "religion, race, or color" is not a consideration for care of the total person. Medicine now is becoming a profession available to all during this era.

The Nuremberg Code was established during the period from 1946 through 1949 as a result of the trials of war criminals following World War II. This code suggests guidelines for human experimentation and is directed to the *world*. It was hoped that the writing of the code would insure the safety of human beings in the years to come.

The Declaration of Helsinki, written during the periods of 1964 through 1975, is an update on human experimentation and much more detailed than the Nuremberg Code. It includes guidelines for both therapeutic and scientific clinical research and also is directed to the *world* of medicine.

Code for Nurses was adopted by the International Council of Nurses in 1973. It is a fairly general code and refers to an idealistic lifestyle and basic standards of nursing care.

The Medical Assistant Code of Ethics is similar to the code of nursing ethics except it is directed to the medical assistant and office and clinic assisting rather than nursing. It was adopted by the American Association of Medical Assistants and appears in its Constitution and Bylaws.

The American Medical Association established the *Principles of Medical Ethics* in 1847, and updated it in 1957 and 1980. The *Preamble* and *Seven Principles* have served as guidelines for physicians, often in great detail as interpreted by the Judicial Council of the AMA, for some time. The Principles are pertinent to physicians and their assistants today.

In the past ten years, other codes have appeared that deal more with the rights of patients than responsibilities and guidelines for health care providers. They include the *Patient's Bill of Rights* presented by the American Hospital Association in 1973. There is a similar bill of rights, *The Pregnant Patient's Bill of Rights,* endorsed by the International Childbirth Education Association. The purpose of such documents has been to inform patients of rights that they have always had but of which they have not always been aware. One of the reasons today for a more-involved laity in medical care is the introduction of such rights.

ETHICAL ISSUES IN MODERN MEDICINE

There are many situations that arise in the practice of medicine and in medical research that present problems requiring moral decisions. A few of these can be illustrated by the following questions.

Should children with serious birth defects be kept alive? Should a woman be allowed an abortion for any reason? Should everyone receive equal treatment in medical care? Should people suffering from a genetic disease be allowed to have children? Should individuals be allowed to die without measures being taken to prolong life/postpone death? Should criteria be developed to determine who receives donor organs?

None of these questions has an easy answer. We probably hope never to have to deal with such questions. There is a possibility, however, that we may sometime be on the receiving end of such decisions or that we may be in positions to assist those who make such decisions. Such questions and possibilities encouraged the inclusion of the following bioethical issues.

There is no attempt in this book to determine right or wrong for the ethical issues in modern medicine. The purpose is to present the facts that are pertinent in the medical office and to raise some questions for consideration. Most of us have decided what "ought" to be in each of the bioethical issues. That is important. It also is important to know how and why our opinions have been formed, and it is necessary to look at what "is," because some of the supports we have felt in the past have fallen away. The "is" of our world must function within the law and within ethical standards.

It is important for us as health professionals to live and act so that we have respect for ourselves and allow others with whom we come in contact to be respected and have respect for themselves, too. We need to know what we are to become; how we can become better than what we are. It is hoped that a discussion of "Allocation of Scarce Medical Resources," "Eugenics," "Artificial Insemination," "Sterilization," "Abortion," "Prolonging Life/Postponing Death by Artificial Means," "Euthanasia," and "Dying and Death" will offer a better understanding of "is" and what may "become." The chapter "Have a Care" and the "Epilogue" will better define for you who we as authors are and what we have become in writing this book.

In reading the following chapters and considering their effect on you personally as well as in your role as a health professional, you may find the following words excerpted from a poem by F. A. Rollo Russel, 1849-1914, helpful.

> Seek the right, perform the true,
> Raise the work and life anew.
> Hearts around you sink with care;
> You can help their load to bear.
> You can bring inspiring light,
> Arm their faltering will to fight.

THE HIPPOCRATIC OATH *

I swear by Apollo Physician and Aslepius and Hygieia and Panaceia and all the gods and goddesses, making them my witnesses, that I will fulfil according to my ability and judgment this oath and this covenant:

To hold him who has taught me this art as equal to my parents and to live my life in partnership with him, and if he is in need of money to give him a share of mine, and to regard his offspring as equal to my brothers in male lineage and to teach them this art—if they desire to learn it—without fee and covenant; to give a share of precepts and oral instruction and all the other learning to my sons and to the sons of him who has instructed me and to pupils who have signed the covenant and have taken an oath according to the medical law, but to no one else.

I will apply dietetic measures for the benefit of the sick according to my ability and judgment; I will keep them from harm and injustice.

I will neither give a deadly drug to anybody if asked for it, nor will I make a suggestion to this effect. Similarly I will not give to a woman an abortive remedy. In purity and holiness I will guard my life and my art.

I will not use the knife, not even on sufferers from stone, but will withdraw in favor of such men as are engaged in this work.

Whatever houses I may visit, I will come for the benefit of the sick, remaining free of all intentional injustice, of all mischief and in particular of sexual relations with both female and male persons, be they free or slaves.

What I may see or hear in the course of the treatment or even outside of the treatment in regard to the life of men, which on no account one must spread abroad, I will keep to myself holding such things shameful to be spoken about.

If I fulfil this oath and do not violate it, may it be granted to me to enjoy life and art, being honored with fame among all men for all time to come; if I transgress it and swear falsely, may the opposite of all this be my lot.

---

*Reprinted with permission of the publisher from "The Hippocratic Oath," in Ludwig Edelstein, *Ancient Medicine*, edited by Oswei Temkin and C. Lillian Temkin (Baltimore: John Hopkins University Press, 1967).

THE GENEVA CONVENTION CODE
OF MEDICAL ETHICS *

I solemnly pledge myself to consecrate my life to the service of humanity;
I will give to my teachers the respect and gratitude which is their due;
I will practice my profession with conscience and dignity;
The health of my patient will be my first consideration;
I will respect the secrets which are confided in me;
I will maintain by all the means in my power, the honour and the noble
    traditions of the medical profession;
My colleagues will be my brothers;
I will not permit considerations of religion, nationality, race, party politics or
    social standing to intervene between my duty and my patient.
I will maintain the utmost respect for human life from the time of concep-
    tion; even under threat. I will not use my medical knowledge contrary
    to the laws of humanity.
I make these promises solemnly, freely and upon my honour.

---

*Reprinted with permission of the World Medical Association. Adopted by the World Medical Association in 1949.

THE NUREMBERG CODE*

The great weight of the evidence before us is to the effect that certain types of medical experiments on human beings, when kept within reasonably well-defined bounds, conform to the ethics of the medical profession generally. The protagonists of the practice of human experimentation justify their views on the basis that such experiments yield results for the good of society that are unprocurable by other methods or means of study. All agree, however, that certain basic principles must be observed in order to satisfy moral, ethical and legal concepts.

1. The voluntary consent of the human subject is absolutely essential.
This means that the person involved should have legal capacity to give consent; should be so situated as to be able to exercise free power of choice, without the intervention of any element of force, fraud, deceit, duress, overreaching, or other ulterior form of constraint or coercion; and should have sufficient knowledge and comprehension of the elements of the subject matter involved as to enable him to make an understanding and enlightened decision. This latter element requires that before the acceptance of an affirmative decision by the experimental subject there should be made known to him the nature, duration, and purpose of the experiment; the method and means by which it is to be conducted; all inconveniences and hazards reasonably to be expected; and the effects upon his health or person which may possibly come from his participation in the experiment.

The duty and responsibility for ascertaining the quality of the consent rests upon each individual who initiates, directs or engages in the experiment. It is a personal duty and responsibility which may not be delegated to another with impunity.

2. The experiment should be such as to yield fruitful results for the good of society, unprocurable by other methods or means of study, and not random and unnecessary in nature.

3. The experiment should be so designed and based on the results of animal experimentation and a knowledge of the natural history of the disease or other problem under study that the anticipated results will justify the performance of the experiment.

4. The experiment should be so conducted as to avoid all unnecessary physical and mental suffering and injury.

5. No experiment should be conducted where there is an *a priori* reason to believe that death or disabling injury will occur; except, perhaps, in those experiments where the experimental physicians also serve as subjects.

---

*From *Trials of War Criminals Before the Nuremberg Military Tribunals Under Control Council Law No. 10*, Vol. II, Nuremberg, October 1946–April 1949.

6. The degree of risk to be taken should never exceed that determined by the humanitarian importance of the problem to be solved by the experiment.

7. Proper preparations should be made and adequate facilities provided to protect the experimental subject against even remote possibilities of injury, disability, or death.

8. The experiment should be conducted only by scientifically qualified persons. The highest degree of skill and care should be required through all stages of the experiment of those who conduct or engage in the experiment.

9. During the course of the experiment the human subject should be at liberty to bring the experiment to an end if he has reached the physical or mental state where continuation of the experiment seems to him to be impossible.

10. During the course of the experiment the scientist in charge must be prepared to terminate the experiment at any stage, if he has probable cause to believe, in the exercise of the good faith, superior skill and careful judgment required of him that a continuation of the experiment is likely to result in injury, disability, or death to the experimental subject.

DECLARATION OF HELSINKI*

Recommendations Guiding Medical Doctors In Biomedical Research Involving Human Services

WORLD MEDICAL ASSOCIATION

Introduction

It is the mission of the medical doctor to safeguard the health of the people. His or her knowledge and conscience are dedicated to the fulfillment of this mission.

The Declaration of Geneva of the World Medical Association binds the doctor with the words, "The health of my patient will be my first consideration;" and the International Code of Medical Ethics declares that, "Any act or advice which could weaken physical or mental resistance of a human being may be used only in his interest."

The purpose of biomedical research involving human subjects must be to improve diagnostic, therapeutic and prophylactic procedures and the understanding of the aetiology and pathogenesis of disease.

In current medical practice most diagnostic, therapeutic or prophylactic procedures involve hazards. This applies *a fortiori* to biomedical research.

Medical progress is based on research which ultimately must rest in part on experimentation involving human subjects.

In the field of biomedical research a fundamental distinction must be recognized between medical research in which the aim is essentially diagnostic or therapeutic for a patient, and medical research, the essential object of which is purely scientific and without direct diagnostic or therapeutic value to the person subjected to the research.

Special caution must be exercised in the conduct of research which may affect the environment, and the welfare of animals used for research must be respected.

Because it is essential that the results of laboratory experiments be applied to human beings to further scientific knowledge and to help suffering humanity, The World Medical Association has prepared the following recommendations as a guide to every doctor in biomedical research involving human subjects. They should be kept under review in the future. It must be stressed that the standards as drafted are only a guide to physicians all over the world. Doctors are not relieved from criminal, civil and ethical responsibilities under the laws of their own countries.

---

*Reprinted with permission of the World Medical Association, Inc., from the "Declaration of Helsinki," revised edition. Adopted by the 18th World Medical Assembly, Helsinki, Finland, 1964, and revised by the 29th World Medical Assembly, Tokyo, Japan, October 1975.

I. Basic Principles

1. Biomedical research involving human subjects must conform to generally accepted scientific principles and should be based on adequately performed laboratory and animal experimentation and on a thorough knowledge of the scientific literature.

2. The design and performance of each experimental procedure involving human subjects should be clearly formulated in an experimental protocol which should be transmitted to a specially appointed independent committee for consideration, comment and guidance.

3. Biomedical research involving human subjects should be conducted only by scientifically qualified persons and under the supervision of a clinically competent medical person. The responsibility for the human subject must always rest with a medically qualified person and never rest on the subject of research, even though the subject has given his or her consent.

4. Biomedical research involving human subjects cannot legitimately be carried out unless the importance of the objective is in proportion to the inherent risk to the subject.

5. Every biomedical research project involving human subjects should be preceded by careful assessment of predictable risks in comparison with foreseeable benefits to the subjects or to others. Concern for the interests of the subject must always prevail over the interests of science and society.

6. The right of the research subject to safeguard his or her integrity must always be respected. Every precaution should be taken to respect the privacy of the subject and to minimize the impact of the study on the subject's physical and mental integrity and on the personality of the subject.

7. Doctors should abstain from engaging in research projects involving human subjects unless they are satisfied that the hazards involved are believed to be predictable. Doctors should cease any investigation if the hazards are found to outweigh the potential benefits.

8. In publication of the results of his or her research, the doctor is obliged to preserve the accuracy of the results. Reports of experimentation not in accordance with the principles laid down in this Declaration should not be accepted for publication.

9. In any research on human beings, each potential subject must be adequately informed of the aims, methods, anticipated benefits and potential hazards of the study and the discomfort it may entail. He or she should be informed that he or she is at liberty to abstain from participation in the study and that he or she is free to withdraw his or her consent to participation at any time. The doctor should then obtain the subject's freely-given informed consent, preferably in writing.

10. When obtaining informed consent for the research project the doctor should be particularly cautious if the subject is in a dependent relationship to him or her or may consent under duress. In that case the

informed consent should be obtained by a doctor who is not engaged in the investigation and who is completely independent of this official relationship.

11. In case of legal incompetence, informed consent should be obtained from the legal guardian in accordance with national legislation. Where physical or mental incapacity makes it impossible to obtain informed consent, or when the subject is a minor, permission from the responsible relative replaces that of the subject in accordance with national legislation.

12. The research protocol should always contain a statement of the ethical considerations involved and should indicate that the principles enunciated in the present Declaration are complied with.

II. Medical Research Combined With Professional Care (Clinical Research)

1. In the treatment of the sick person, the doctor must be free to use a new diagnostic and therapeutic measure, if in his or her judgement it offers hope of saving life, reestablishing health or alleviating suffering.

2. The potential benefits, hazards and discomfort of a new method should be weighed against the advantages of the best current diagnostic and therapeutic methods.

3. In any medical study, every patient—including those of a control group, if any—should be assured of the best proven diagnostic and therapeutic method.

4. The refusal of the patient to participate in a study must never interfere with the doctor-patient relationship.

5. If the doctor considers it essential not to obtain informed consent, the specific reasons for this proposal should be stated in the experimental protocol for transmission to the independent committee (I, 2).

6. The doctor can combine medical research with professional care, the objective being the acquisition of new medical knowledge, only to the extent that medical research is justified by its potential diagnostic or therapeutic value for the patient.

III. Non-Therapeutic Biomedical Research Involving Human Subjects (Non-Clinical Biomedical Research)

1. In the purely scientific application of medical research carried out on a human being, it is the duty of the doctor to remain the protector of life and health of that person on whom biomedical research is being carried out.

2. The subjects should be volunteers—either healthy persons or patients for whom the experimental design is not related to the patient's illness.

3. The investigator or the investigating team should discontinue the research if in his/her or their judgement it may, if continued, be harmful to the individual.

4. In research on man, the <u>interest of science and society should</u> <u>never take precedence</u> over <u>considerations related to the well-being of the</u> <u>subject</u>.

CODE FOR NURSES*

ETHICAL CONCEPTS APPLIED TO NURSING

The fundamental responsibility of the nurse is fourfold: to promote health, to prevent illness, to restore health and to alleviate suffering.

The need for nursing is universal. Inherent in nursing is respect for life, dignity and rights of man. It is unrestricted by considerations of nationality, race, creed, colour, age, sex, politics or social status.

Nurses render health services to the individual, the family and the community and coordinate their services with those of related groups.

Nurses and People

The nurse's primary responsibility is to those people who require nursing care.

The nurse, in providing care, promotes an environment in which the values, customs and spiritual beliefs of the individual are respected.

The nurse holds in confidence personal information and uses judgement in sharing this information.

Nurses and Practice

The nurse carries personal responsibility for nursing practice and for maintaining competence by continual learning.

The nurse maintains the highest standards of nursing care possible within the reality of a specific situation.

The nurse uses judgement in relation to individual competence when accepting and delegating responsibilities.

The nurse when acting in a professional capacity should at all times maintain standards of personal conduct which reflect credit upon the profession.

Nurses and Society

The nurse shares with other citizens the responsibility for initiating and supporting action to meet the health and social needs of the public.

Nurses and Co-Workers

The nurse sustains a cooperative relationship with co-workers in nursing and other fields.

---

*Reprinted with permission of the International Council of Nurses, Geneva, Switzerland. The Code for Nurses, as printed here, was produced by the Professional Services Committee and adopted by the ICN Council of National Representatives in Mexico City in May 1973.

The nurse takes appropriate action to safeguard the individual when his care is endangered by a co-worker or any other person.

Nurses and the Profession

The nurse plays the major role in determining and implementing desirable standards of nursing practice and nursing education.

The nurse is active in developing a core of professional knowledge.

The nurse, acting through the professional organization, participates in establishing and maintaining equitable social and economic working conditions in nursing.

CODE OF ETHICS

AMERICAN ASSOCIATION OF MEDICAL ASSISTANTS*

The Code of Ethics of AAMA shall set forth principles of ethical and moral conduct as they relate to the medical profession and the particular practice of medical assisting.

Members of AAMA dedicated to the conscientious pursuit of their profession, and thus desiring to merit the high regard of the entire medical profession and the respect of the general public which they serve, do pledge themselves to strive always to:

A. render service with full respect for the dignity of humanity;
B. respect confidential information obtained through employment unless legally authorized or required by responsible performance of duty to divulge such information;
C. uphold the honor and high principles of the profession and accept its disciplines;
D. seek to continually improve the knowledge and skills of medical assistants for the benefit of patients and professional colleagues;
E. participate in additional service activities aimed toward improving the health and well-being of the community.

CREED

I believe in the principles and purposes of the profession of medical assisting.

I endeavor to be more effective.

I aspire to render greater service.

I protect the confidence entrusted to me.

I am dedicated to the care and well-being of all patients.

I am loyal to my physician-employer.

I am true to the ethics of my profession.

I am strengthened by compassion, courage, and faith.

*Printed with permission of the American Association of Medical Assistants, Inc. *Bylaws*, American Association of Medical Assistants. Adopted October 1980.

PRINCIPLES OF MEDICAL ETHICS

AMERICAN MEDICAL ASSOCIATION*

PREAMBLE:

The medical profession has long subscribed to a body of ethical statements developed primarily for the benefit of the patient. As a member of this profession, a physician must recognize responsibility not only to patients, but also to society, to other health professionals, and to self. The following Principles adopted by the American Medical Association are not laws, but standards of conduct which define the essentials of honorable behavior for the physician.

I.   A physician shall be dedicated to providing competent medical service with compassion and respect for human dignity.

II. A physician shall deal honestly with patients and colleagues, and strive to expose those physicians deficient in character or competence, or who engage in fraud or deception.

III. A physician shall respect the law and also recognize a responsibility to seek changes in those requirements which are contrary to the best interests of the patient.

IV. A physician shall respect the rights of patients, of colleagues, and of other health professionals, and shall safeguard patient confidences within the constraints of the law.

V.   A physician shall continue to study, apply and advance scientific knowledge, make relevant information available to patients, colleagues, and the public, obtain consultation, and use the talents of other health professionals when indicated.

VI. A physician shall, in the provision of appropriate patient care, except in emergencies, be free to choose whom to serve, with whom to associate, and the environment in which to provide medical services.

VII. A physician shall recognize a responsibility to participate in activities contributing to an improved community.

*Printed with permission of the American Medical Association. Adopted August 1980. (DAD:80-904 20M:8/80)

A PATIENT'S BILL OF RIGHTS

AMERICAN HOSPITAL ASSOCIATION*

The American Hospital Association Board of Trustees' Committee on Health Care for the Disadvantaged, which has been a consistent advocate on behalf of consumers of health care services, developed the Statement on a Patient's Bill of Rights, which was approved by the AHA House of Delegates February 6, 1973. The statement was published in several forms, one of which was the S74 leaflet in the Association's S series. The S74 leaflet is now superseded by this reprinting of the statement.

The American Hospital Association presents a Patient's Bill of Rights with the expectation that observance of these rights will contribute to more effective patient care and greater satisfaction for the patient, his physician, and the hospital organization. Further, the Association presents these rights in the expectation that they will be supported by the hospital on behalf of its patients, as an integral part of the healing process. It is recognized that a personal relationship between the physician and the patient is essential for the provision of proper medical care. The traditional physician-patient relationship takes on a new dimension when care is rendered within an organizational structure. Legal precedent has established that the institution itself also has a responsibility to the patient. It is in recognition of these factors that these rights are affirmed.

1. The patient has the right to considerate and respectful care.

2. The patient has the right to obtain from his physician complete current information concerning his diagnosis, treatment, and prognosis in terms the patient can be reasonably expected to understand. When it is not medically advisable to give such information to the patient, the information should be made available to an appropriate person in his behalf. He has the right to know, by name, the physician responsible for coordinating his care.

3. The patient has the right to receive from his physician information necessary to give informed consent prior to the start of any procedure and/or treatment. Except in emergencies, such information for informed consent should include but not necessarily be limited to the specific procedure and/or treatment, the medically significant risks involved, and the probable duration of incapacitation. Where medically significant alternatives for care or treatment exist, or when the patient requests information concerning medical alternatives, the patient has the right to such information. The patient also has the right to know the name of the person responsible for the procedures and/or treatment.

---

*Reprinted with the permission of the American Hospital Association, Copyright 1975.

4. The patient has the right to refuse treatment to the extent permitted by law and to be informed of the medical consequences of his action.

5. The patient has the right to every consideration of his privacy concerning his own medical care program. Case discussion, consultation, examination, and treatment are confidential and should be conducted discreetly. Those not directly involved in his care must have the permission of the patient to be present.

6. The patient has the right to expect that all communications and records pertaining to his care should be treated as confidential.

7. The patient has the right to expect that within its capacity a hospital must make reasonable response to the request of a patient for services. The hospital must provide evaluation, service, and/or referral as indicated by the urgency of the case. When medically permissible, a patient may be transferred to another facility only after he has received complete information and explanation concerning the needs for and alternatives to such a transfer. The institution to which the patient is to be transferred must first have accepted the patient for transfer.

8. The patient has the right to obtain information as to any relationship of his hospital to other health care and educational institutions insofar as his care is concerned. The patient has the right to obtain information as to the existence of any professional relationships among individuals, by name, who are treating him.

9. The patient has the right to be advised if the hospital proposes to engage in or perform human experimentation affecting his care or treatment. The patient has the right to refuse to participate in such research projects.

10. The patient has the right to expect reasonable continuity of care. He has the right to know in advance what appointment times and physicians are available and where. The patient has the right to expect that the hospital will provide a mechanism whereby he is informed by his physician or a delegate of the physician of the patient's continuing health care requirements following discharge.

11. The patient has the right to examine and receive an explanation of his bill regardless of source of payment.

12. The patient has the right to know what hospital rules and regulations apply to his conduct as a patient.

No catalog of rights can guarantee for the patient the kind of treatment he has a right to expect. A hospital has many functions to perform, including the prevention and treatment of disease, the education of both health professionals and patients, and the conduct of clinical research. All these activities must be conducted with an overriding concern for the patient, and, above all, the recognition of his dignity as a human being. Success in achieving this recognition assures success in the defense of the rights of the patient.

THE PREGNANT PATIENT'S BILL OF RIGHTS*

American parents are becoming increasingly aware that well-intentioned health professionals do not always have scientific data to support common American obstetrical practices and that many of these practices are carried out primarily because they are part of medical and hospital tradition. In the last forty years many artificial practices have been introduced which have changed childbirth from a physiological event to a very complicated medical procedure in which all kinds of drugs are used and procedures carried out, sometimes unnecessarily, and many of them potentially damaging for the baby and even for the mother. A growing body of research makes it alarmingly clear that every aspect of traditional American hospital care during labor and delivery must now be questioned as to its possible effect on the future well-being of both the obstetric patient and her unborn child.

One in every 35 children born in the United States today will eventually be diagnosed as retarded; in 75% of these cases there is no familial or genetic predisposing factor. One in every 10 to 17 children has been found to have some form of brain dysfunction or learning disability requiring special treatment. Such statistics are not confined to the lower socioeconomic group but cut across all segments of American society.

New concerns are being raised by childbearing women because no one knows what degree of oxygen depletion, head compression, or traction by forceps the unborn or newborn infant can tolerate before that child sustains permanent brain damage or dysfunction. The recent findings regarding the cancer-related drug diethylstilbestrol have alerted the public to the fact that neither the approval of a drug by the U.S. Food and Drug Administration nor the fact that a drug is prescribed by a physician serves as a guarantee that a drug or medication is safe for the mother or her unborn child. In fact, the American Academy of Pediatrics' Committee on Drugs has recently stated that there is no drug, whether prescription or over-the-counter remedy, which has been proven safe for the unborn child.

The Pregnant Patient has the right to participate in decisions involving her well-being and that of her unborn child, unless there is a clearcut medical emergency that prevents her participation. In addition to the rights set forth in the American Hospital Association's "Patient's Bill of Rights," (which has also been adopted by the New York City Department of Health) the Pregnant Patient, because she represents TWO patients rather than one, should be recognized as having the additional rights listed below.

1. *The Pregnant Patient has the right,* prior to the administration of any drug or procedure, to be informed by the health professional caring for her

---

*Reprinted with permission from the International Childbirth Education Association, Inc. Prepared by Doris Haire, Chair., ICEA Committee on Health Law and Regulation.

of any potential direct or indirect effects, risks or hazards to herself or her unborn or newborn infant which may result from the use of a drug or procedure prescribed for or administered to her during pregnancy, labor, birth or lactation.

2. *The Pregnant Patient has the right,* prior to the proposed therapy, to be informed, not only of the benefits, risks and hazards of the proposed therapy but also of known alternative therapy, such as available childbirth education classes which could help to prepare the Pregnant Patient physically and mentally to cope with the discomfort or stress of pregnancy and the experience of childbirth, thereby reducing or eliminating her need for drugs and obstetric intervention. She should be offered such information early in her pregnancy in order that she may make a reasoned decision.

3. *The Pregnant Patient has the right,* prior to the administration of any drug, to be informed by the health professional who is prescribing or administering the drug to her that any drug which she receives during pregnancy, labor and birth, no matter how or when the drug is taken or administered, may adversely affect her unborn baby, directly or indirectly, and that there is no drug or chemical which has been proven safe for the unborn child.

4. *The Pregnant Patient has the right* if Cesarean birth is anticipated, to be informed prior to the administration of any drug, and preferably prior to her hospitalization, that minimizing her and, in turn, her baby's intake of nonessential pre-operative medicine will benefit her baby.

5. *The Pregnant Patient has the right,* prior to the administration of a drug or procedure, to be informed of the areas of uncertainty if there is NO properly controlled follow-up research which has established the safety of the drug or procedure with regard to its direct and/or indirect effects on the physiological, mental and neurological development of the child exposed, via the mother, to the drug or procedure during pregnancy, labor, birth or lactation—(this would apply to virtually all drugs and the vast majority of obstetric procedures).

6. *The Pregnant Patient has the right,* prior to the administration of any drug, to be informed of the brand name and generic name of the drug in order that she may advise the health professional of any past adverse reaction to the drug.

7. *The Pregnant Patient has the right* to determine for herself, without pressure from her attendant, whether she will accept the risks inherent in the proposed therapy or refuse a drug or procedure.

8. *The Pregnant Patient has the right* to know the name and qualifications of the individual administering a medication or procedure to her during labor or birth.

9. *The Pregnant Patient has the right* to be informed, prior to the administration of any procedure, whether that procedure is being administered to her for her or her baby's benefit (medically indicated) or as an elective procedure (for convenience, teaching purposes or research).

10. *The Pregnant Patient has the right* to be accompanied during the stress of labor and birth by someone she cares for, and to whom she looks for emotional comfort and encouragement.

11. *The Pregnant Patient* has the right after appropriate medical consultation to choose a position for labor and for birth which is least stressful to her baby and to herself.

12. *The Obstetric Patient* has the right to have her baby cared for at her bedside if her baby is normal, and to feed her baby according to her baby's needs rather than according to the hospital regimen.

13. *The Obstetric Patient has the right* to be informed in writing of the name of the person who actually delivered her baby and the professional qualifications of that person. This information should also be on the birth certificate.

14. *The Obstetric Patient has the right* to be informed if there is any known or indicated aspect of her or her baby's care or condition which may cause her or her baby later difficulty or problems.

15. *The Obstetric Patient has the right* to have her and her baby's hospital medical records complete, accurate and legible and to have their records, including Nurses' Notes, retained by the hospital until the child reaches the age of majority, or, alternatively, to have the records offered to her before they are destroyed.

16. *The Obstetric Patient,* both during and after her hospital stay, has the right to have access to her complete hospital medical records, including Nurses' Notes, and to receive a copy upon payment of a reasonable fee and without incurring the expense of retaining an attorney.

It is the obstetric patient and her baby, not the health professional, who must sustain any trauma or injury resulting from the use of a drug or obstetric procedure. The observation of the rights listed above will not only permit the obstetric patient to participate in the decisions involving her and her baby's health care, but will help to protect the health professional and the hospital against litigation arising from resentment or misunderstanding on the part of the mother.

REFERENCES

1.	VAUX, K: *Biomedical Ethics.* Harper and Row, New York, 1974, pp xii-xiii.

DISCUSSION QUESTIONS

1. What is the difference between law and ethics? Can a law be unethical? Can an ethic be unlawful?

2. What would you do if your ethics do not agree with your physician-employer's?

3. Why is an understanding of bioethics important?

4. Do the Medical Assistant Code of Ethics and the Principles of Medical Ethics have any conflicting views?

CHAPTER 12

ALLOCATION OF
SCARCE MEDICAL RESOURCES

LEARNING OBJECTIVES

Upon successful completion of this chapter, you will:

1. Define *macro*allocation of scarce resources.

2. Describe how decisions are made at the *macro*allocation level.

3. Define *micro*allocation of scarce resources.

4. Describe how decisions are made at the *micro*allocation level.

5. Describe both systems of selection.

DEFINITIONS

Bioethics. Morals or ethics connected with biology or medicine.

Eugenics. Improvement of a race by the control of human procreation.

Macroallocation. System in which distribution decisions are made by large bodies of individuals, usually Congress, Health Systems Agencies, state legislatures, health insurance companies.

Microallocation. System in which distribution decisions are made by small groups and/or individuals such as hospital staff and physicians.

INTRODUCTION

You are employed for a team of transplant surgeons in a major city when a call comes from a hospital that donor organs are available. The wheels move quickly to determine proper matches among the clinic's patients. Your physicians discover that two equally needy patients surface for the donor liver. How is a decision made?

A young boy in a very rural area of the country dies in a hospital following an automobile accident. Your physician, on emergency call at the hospital when the ambulance brings in the patient, works feverishly for over an hour, but the boy dies. Your physician relates to you the next morning the feeling of hopelessness knowing the boy's life might have been saved if a neurosurgeon and more sophisticated equipment had been accessible to the hospital. How is it that geographical location may dictate who lives and who dies?

The family at 913 Twelfth Street will be saved from financial ruin because Medicare will help defray the costs of their young son's kidney dialysis. But the family at 909 Twelfth Street may suffer great financial stress due to the increasing medical bills caused by their daughter's juvenile-onset diabetes mellitus, which already requires laser treatments for retinopathy in her eyes. How does a government determine one medical problem warrants financial assistance and another does not?

Should two hospitals in the same city have a CAT scanner? Must each have every piece of the latest equipment or diagnostic device? Would it be wise to encourage each hospital to develop a "specialty" in areas of treatment rather than a duplication? Would such a plan assure the patient the "best possible care?"

These questions are not easy for anyone to answer. There may not be any "right" or "wrong" answers. As an employee in the medical office, you may never come in direct contact with these situations, but they are matters dealt with on a daily basis.

The problem presented by these questions is both economical and ethical. The economical question is, "How can scarce resources be allocated in light of costs required and still satisfy human needs and/or desires?" The ethical question is, "How will these scarce resources be justly and fairly distributed?"[1]

Health professionals, researchers, and members of nearly all academic disciplines have been formally discussing such issues for almost a decade. These individuals further define the problem in terms of *macro*allocation and *micro*allocation of scarce resources.[2]

MACROALLOCATION AND MICROALLOCATION

Macroallocation decisions are made concerning *how much* shall be expended for medical resources as well as how they are to be distributed. These decisions are made by larger bodies, such as Congress, Health Systems Agencies, state legislatures, health organizations, private foundations, and health insurance companies. For example, it was Congress that determined Medicare should provide medical care for the chronic renal patient. No other chronic disease is specifically named in the Medicare program. Macroallocation decisions also are evident when determinations are made regarding funding of medical research. How much should be allotted for cancer research, for preventive medicine, or for expensive equipment? The health insurance industry largely determines the "reasonable and customary" charges in medical care and what will and will not be covered by health insurance premiums.[3]

*Micro*allocation decisions are made on an individual basis, usually by local hospital policy and doctors concerning *who shall* obtain the resources available. Decisions at the microallocation level cut deeper into our consciousness, because it is a little like asking, "Who shall live when not everyone can live?"[4] Such examples requiring these decisions include hemodialysis machines and organs donated for transplantation. Who is allowed to occupy the one available bed in intensive care? Does the Medicaid patient receive the same care as the local VIP?

SYSTEMS FOR DECISION-MAKING

How are the criteria that attempt to answer such questions established? Two prominent systems have arisen. One system identifies three possible selection processes. The second system identifies five principles for a fair selection process. The two are outlined below.

SYSTEM I—Three positions of selection

1. *Combination Criteria Systems* Those who satisfy the most criteria ought to receive treatment. Such criteria might include (a) capacity to benefit from treatment without complications, (b) ability to contribute financially or experimentally as a research subject, (c) age and life expectancy, and (d) past and potential future contributions of the patient to society.
2. *Random Selection Systems* This system is more like "first come, first served," or a simple chance selection or drawing of lots.
3. *No-Treatment Systems* This system is based on the premise that if all cannot be treated, then treatment should be given to none.[5]

SYSTEM II—Five positions of selection

Decisions should be made on the following bases:

1. To everyone an equal share.
2. To everyone according to their individual needs.
3. To everyone according to their individual efforts.

4. To everyone according to their contributions to society.
5. To everyone according to their abilities and merits.[6]

It should be obvious to the reader at this point that no established criteria present a final solution to the problem. None would be easy to follow. Factors other than those mentioned in the two systems will also influence decisions. They include personal ethics, personal preferences, religion, geographical location, and the political climate. Many problems and few solutions are evident when considering how and to whom scarce medical resources should be allocated. This bioethical issue is complex, but is one the allied health professional cannot ignore, as it will present itself frequently.

HEALTH SYSTEMS AGENCY

In the United States an attempt is being made to address the issue of allocation of medical resources through the Health Systems Agency. In 1974 Congress enacted the National Health Planning and Resources Development Act (Public Law 93-641)[7] the overall goal of which is to achieve "equal access to quality health care at a reasonable cost . . ."

Public Law 93-641 spells out national health goals and priorities:

Major Goals

1. To improve health.
2. To increase accessibility and quality of health services.
3. To restrain costs.
4. To prevent unnecessary duplication of health resources.

Major Priorities

1. An emphasis on primary care services for the medically underserved.
2. Coordination and consolidation of hospital services.
3. Wide use of health education to improve personal health care and to explain how to use the health system.
4. Promotion of preventive health care.

NATIONAL PLANS

Implementation of the goals occurs at national and state levels. Some state plans include subarea councils. The national plan is as follows:

National Health Advisory Council

1. Is appointed by the Secretary of the Department of Health and Human Services (HHS).
2. Develops recommendations on health policy to HHS, to the Congress, and to the nation.

U.S. Department of Health and Human Services

1. Administers Public Law 93-641 through the Health Resources Administration of the Public Health Service.
2. Designates health systems agencies and state health planning and development agencies.
3. Approves and funds health planning programs of health systems agencies and state health planning and development agencies.

STATE PLANS

State agencies begin when the governor appoints the State Health Coordinating Council (SHCC). This Council develops statewide health policies and coordinates the plans of the Health Systems Agencies, also designated by the governor.

State Health Planning and Development Agency (State Agency)

1. Administers, through the State Department of Social and Health Services, the state health program.
2. Prepares a preliminary State Health Plan consolidating the plans of the health systems agencies and submits the SHP to the State Health Coordinating Council for approval.
3. Makes decisions about granting Certificates of Need, state permits for construction, equipment purchase, or remodeling projects in excess of $150,000 for hospitals and nursing homes.

Health Systems Agency (HSA)

1. Is designated by the Secretary of HHS to serve the health service area designated by the governor.
2. Conducts health planning within its area.
3. May be a private nonprofit or a public organization.
4. Performs specific functions outlined in Public Law 93-641.
5. Must have qualified staff.
6. May include subarea councils.

Subarea councils allow input at a level closest to the actual health care consumer. States will differ in the number of Health Systems Agencies and where there are subarea councils.

Public Law 93-641 is an attempt by Congress to determine the allocation of our scarce medical resources. This is considered *macro*allocation. As with any organization of this size, the main purpose can be easily buried in the political bureaucracy which develops. Implementation of the law also is dependent upon available funding, which is not guaranteed by the federal government.

REFERENCES

1. BEAUCHAMP, TL AND WALTERS, L: *Contemporary Issues in Bioethics*. Dickinson, Belmont, CA, 1978, p 347.
2. IBID, pp 348-349.
3. IBID, p 347.
4. IBID, p 349.
5. IBID, p 350.
6. IBID, p 348.
7. *Some Background on PSHSA*. Puget Sound Health Systems Agency, Seattle, WA, 1981, pp 1-9.

DISCUSSION QUESTIONS

1. Consider each of the examples at the beginning of the chapter and answer the following questions:
    1. At what level (*macro*allocation or *micro*allocation) is a decision made?
    2. Can one of the selection systems be applied?

2. Who is allowed to occupy the *one* bed in intensive care? How is a decision made?

3. On what basis do you decide who gets the very last open slot of the physician's appointment book? What system of selection is followed?

4. Two patients desperately need the use of one remaining hemodialysis machine. One is aged and a Medicaid patient. The other is a young college student who has full health insurance benefits. Who decides? Support your answer.

5. Dr. Progressive is denied a Certificate of Need for the fully equipped laboratory that is requested. The doctor feels the decision may have been influenced by the local hospital administrator, who prefers that all physicians in the area utilize the services of the hospital laboratory. Discuss.

CHAPTER **13**

EUGENICS

LEARNING OBJECTIVES

Upon successful completion of this chapter, you will:

1. Define negative and positive eugenics and cite a sample of each.
2. Name at least six diseases to be determined by genetic testing.
3. Compare voluntary and mandatory genetic screening.
4. Describe in-vitro fertilization, listing its advantages and disadvantages.
5. Explain cloning as a form of eugenics.
6. Describe how amniocentesis is used in genetic testing.
7. Recall two indicators of amniocentesis and two possible outcomes.
8. List four problems encountered in determining "who decides?"
9. Identify two major legal implications to eugenics.

DEFINITIONS

Amniocentesis. Method of prenatal diagnosis in which a needle is used to withdraw fluid from the amniotic sac within the uterus of a pregnant woman.

Asexual. Without sex; no sexual intercourse.

Artificial Insemination. Instrumental introduction of semen into the vagina so that the woman may conceive.

Blastocyst. An early embryonic cluster of cells that attaches to the uterus wall and develops into the actual embryo.

Cloning. Asexual method of producing offspring; genetically identical to the parent cell.

Cystic Fibrosis. Hereditary disease affecting the pancreas, lungs, and sweat glands, causing chronic respiratory infection, pancreatic insufficiency, and heat intolerance. Prognosis is poor; no cure.

Down's Syndrome. Also called mongolism; condition resulting from chromosomal abnormality causing moderate-to-severe mental retardation.

Eugenics. The improvement of a race by the control of human procreation.

Hemophilia. Hereditary disease characterized by poor clotting ability; occurs almost exclusively in males; no known cure; bleeder's disease.

Negative Eugenics. A type of eugenics aimed at decreasing the number of undesirable or harmful genes.

Phenylketonuria (PKU). Hereditary disease due to an enzyme deficiency; if treatment of special diet is started early in infancy, prognosis is good; if untreated, brain damage results.

Positive Eugenics. A type of eugenics aimed at increasing the number of favorable genes in the human population.

Sex-Linked. Transmitted by a gene located on an X or Y (sex) chromosome.

Sickle-Cell Anemia. Hereditary, chronic form of anemia, affecting principally people of Negro populations.

Spina Bifida. Congenital disease characterized by part of the spinal cord and its coverings being exposed through a gap in the backbone, forming a tumor known as spina bifida.

Surrogate. Substitute; someone or something replacing another.

Tay-Sachs Disease. Hereditary disease causing degeneration of the nervous system characterized by mental and physical retardation, and blindness. No treatment; prognosis is poor with death usually occurring within the first two to three years of life. Occurs almost exclusively among people of Jewish descent.

Ultrasound. Sound waves of extremely high frequency used to examine structures inside the body for diagnostic purposes.

INTRODUCTION

Nineteenth- and twentieth-century developments in science give rise to moral and social issues of considerable complexity. One of the more complex issues is *eugenics*—the improvement of a race by the control of human procreation. There are two points of view of eugenics—*positive eugenics* and *negative eugenics*.

Positive eugenics aims at *increasing* the number of favorable genes in the human population. This premise favors social policies and practices that increase the number of genes in the human population responsible for *improving* traits that we value, such as intelligence.

Negative eugenics aims at decreasing the number of *undesirable* or harmful genes. This premise advocates eliminating or reducing the number of those genes that are responsible for various kinds of birth defects and sex-linked diseases.[1]

Both positive and negative eugenics require instituting some kind of control over human reproduction. Some procedures and possibilities related to this issue are considered.

GENETIC TESTING AND GENETIC SCREENING

Over 2,000 genetically related disorders have been identified. In some cases, genetic testing is helpful in treating a patient's disorder. In others, no treatment or cure is possible even if genetic testing can detect the "carriers" of many disorders as well as the "sufferers."

Genetic testing and screening had its beginnings as a *voluntary* measure to discover persons already suffering from a particular disease. (An example is phenylketonuria [PKU].) The second development was the institution of *mandatory* testing. (In most states PKU testing is now mandatory for all newborns.) The latest stage in the development seeks to detect the *carriers* as well as the *sufferers* of particular genetic diseases. (Some states require screening for carriers of sickle-cell trait.)[2] This latter stage brings us face to face with eugenics.

Through genetic testing and screening, a number of genetic diseases can be predicted with a certain degree of probability. Such diseases are hemophilia, Tay-Sachs disease, sickle-cell anemia, Down's syndrome, and phenylketonuria.

The proponent of negative eugenics might advocate that a screening process for *all* detectable genetic diseases be required by law. Potential sufferers could be encouraged to have no children. There are no laws that make it a crime for genetically "bad risk" individuals to have children, but we may be moving closer to that regulation. Several states now require the screening of newborn infants to detect certain genetic diseases (such as PKU) that respond to early treatment. Also, some states require that applicants for marriage licenses be tested for the presence of sickle-cell trait, and no states allow the marriage of first cousins. This illustrates the movement of screening from voluntary to mandatory.

Genetic counseling is generally voluntary. Its purpose is to provide information rather than to dictate decisions on reproduction. Its goal is to decrease the number of children suffering from birth defects and genetic diseases. However, such counseling can discourage the birth of children carrying harmful genes. This, in turn, discourages the spread of those genes in the human population. It also is possible that such counseling could be used to encourage those couples with favorable genes to produce large numbers of children.

To further illustrate the complexity of eugenics, consider the following situations and the possible ethical and legal ramifications.

A 45-year-old expectant mother of six is requesting amniocentesis to determine Down's syndrome. In an adjacent exam room a young woman experiencing her first pregnancy also is concerned about Down's syndrome. Her sister is afflicted with the disease, and knowing the tendency can be familial, she also requests amniocentesis. Will the genetic counseling of each woman differ? Support your answer. Each woman asks you, "What would you do in my situation?"

IN-VITRO FERTILIZATION AND CLONING

A rather recent development in eugenics is *in-vitro fertilization*—literally, fertilization in glass. In-vitro fertilization is the process of fertilizing the ovum "in glass," allowing it to multiply and divide, and then implanting it into the uterus. This technique has been accomplished successfully in several species of animals. Animal breeders have been selectively altering the composition of genetic organisms for many years.[3] Successful test-tube fertilization and embryo transfer in humans was achieved in the early 1980s. Currently, only a few children have been born as the result of in-vitro fertilization. Many geneticists believe there are other successful "test-tube babies" whose identities have been kept secret.

Among the potential benefits of in-vitro fertilization is that it will allow many women who are infertile because of blocked fallopian tubes or oviducts to bear children. This is done by removing the ovum from the potential mother and placing it in a dish containing blood serum and nutrients. Sperm is added. Once an egg is fertilized, it then is transferred to another dish where, for the next three to six days, the fertilized egg divides, creating a cluster of cells called a blastocyst. The blastocyst is placed in the uterus, where it is attached to the wall and normal development proceeds.[4]

Eugenics plays a more complex role if the semen is other than the husband's (artificial insemination) or a surrogate (substitute) mother is used. A surrogate mother is one who donates her ovum and who agrees to carry the unborn for the prospective parent(s) until its birth. At that time, the infant is given up by the surrogate mother. Either surrogating or artificial insemination automatically implies careful selectivity in the reproduction process. It also can raise delicate legal questions regarding parentage of the offspring—questions not yet addressed by most states. These problems occur when either the donor of semen or the surrogate mother chooses not to relinquish rights to the unborn. Surrogate mothers may find it very difficult to relinquish all rights to a child they have carried for nine months of pregnancy. Because the identity of surrogate mothers and donors of semen is usually kept confidential, it does raise, however, the long-term possibility of marriage between unknowing half-brothers or sisters.

Cloning is the term used to refer to a method of producing offspring asexually. Unlike sexual reproduction, which combines genetic material from two individuals and produces offspring uniquely different from either, asexual reproduction, or cloning, results in offspring produced asexually and identical to a single cell.

Clonal frogs have successfully been produced, and some scientists predict that a clonal human being, however more complex the process, will be produced in the early 2100s. Other scientists believe a human being will never be cloned due to resistance from society. The cloning of human beings would certainly remove the "chance" inherent in human reproduction as it exists now. Other possibilities include predetermination of gender, preservation of individuals with special capabilities useful to society, and preservation of family likenesses. All genetic diseases could be eliminated through selective cloning. Intelligence and beauty could be guaranteed to every offspring. However, the asexually produced child would suffer from the lack of the natural bond that exists between parents and their children. Individual uniqueness, valued so much in our society, would soon become rare if humans were cloned.[5]

Cloning is one aspect of eugenics to be explored. The complexity of human biology, the fact that no mammal has yet been cloned, and society's resistance to the process places cloning human beings far in the future.

In the normal sex cell there are 23 chromosomes. When the human sperm and ovum unite, there are a total of 46 chromosomes, half from the female and half from the male. In cloning, the nucleus would be removed from the female ovum and a body cell from another human (containing all 46 chromosomes) would be implanted in that ovum.

If the egg were then embedded in the uterus, and it grew to maturity, a human being would then exist with the same genetic make-up as the person who donated the body cell.[6]

AMNIOCENTESIS—DETERMINING DISEASE, MALFORMATION, SEX

A subject related to eugenics that is far more familiar to the medical office employee is *amniocentesis*. Amniocentesis is the removal of fluid from the amniotic cavity by needle puncture.

A sample of fluid surrounding the fetus is taken by inserting a sterile needle into the amniotic cavity and withdrawing a small amount of fluid.

This fluid, containing fetal cells, is centrifuged to separate the cells from fluid. The cells then are studied for genetic defects. The best time for amniocentesis for genetic diagnosis is about the 16th week of gestation.[7]

Ultrasound is used in conjunction with amniocentesis for placement of the needle for amniocentesis. Ultrasound is used to examine structure inside the body, much the same as x-rays, but with the advantage the patient is not submitted to harmful radiation. Ultrasound is sound waves of extremely high frequency inaudible to the human ear. It is comparable to sonar systems used by submarines to find underwater objects. Sound waves are bounced off an object, producing a photograph.

Among the 40 or more genetic diseases to be determined by tests on the amniotic fluid and its cells are cystic fibrosis, Down's syndrome, and sickle-cell anemia. Several referral centers throughout the country have facilities to perform all these tests.[8] The results of the tests and the genetic counseling have far-reaching effects on us as individuals and on society as a whole.

The most obvious purpose of such testing is to determine genetic diseases that would cause suffering and/or death to the offspring as well as an emotional burden on parents. There are currently two clear indicators to health professionals for amniocentesis. One is advanced maternal age, which greatly increases the risk of Down's syndrome. The second is a pregnancy of a woman who has previously borne a child with a genetic disease.[9] The outcome is also twofold. One outcome informs prospective parents of the difficulty so they may be better prepared to face the problem at the time of birth and in the future. The second outcome is the practice of selective abortion.

Neither outcome is an easy solution to a genetic disease, especially since the mother is already well into the pregnancy. Selective abortion at that time can be a traumatic experience. All kinds of questions surface to the patient who discovers a genetic disease through amniocentesis. Can I or the child live with the disease? How long? How "normal" will our lives be? What financial obligations will this have on the family? How will siblings be affected? Do I have a right to choose an abortion? Does the child have a right to life only or a right to a healthy, normal existence free from pain, agony, and deformity? Who decides? On what basis is a decision made?

Another result of amniocentesis is that the sex of the unborn can be determined. While this may serve only as a convenience to parents planning for the birth, there are geneticists who warn that some may choose selective abortion on the basis of sex only. Before making the statement, "I don't believe eugenics will ever come to that," consider the number of cultures in our world that prefer the male offspring to the female. While the plea of the 1980s has been for "human rights," there is at least one country in our world that has a declining female population (contrary to what is known about population statistics).

WHO DECIDES

The greatest question for eugenics is "Who decides?" Do governments mandate that genetic screening be performed on all individuals? Should genetic counseling be required of all, much the same as a blood test may be a requirement for a marriage license? Should in-vitro fertilization be encouraged for infertile parents only, or should it be available to any who desire it? Should additional federal funds be released for genetic research to encourage the possibility of a healthier existence for all? Is it possible that other countries more advanced in genetic research than the United States will be able to produce a superior race through cloning? Should negative eugenics, such as occurred between 1911 and 1930 when 33 states passed the laws requiring sterilization for a variety of "undesirable" behavioral traits, be encouraged or discouraged?[10] Who decides what is a desirable or undesirable behavioral trait? Would it be based solely on IQ or on the amount of public funds that might be required to support a person of "undesirable" traits?

Few health professionals are willing to make a statement on "who decides" openly and freely. Yet such decisions are being made daily. Decisions in the realm of eugenics are going to become more difficult as time passes. Physicians and employees need to be sensitive and responsive to the needs of patients.

LEGAL IMPLICATIONS

Generally, the *major* legal implication of the eugenics topics is the informed consent of all involved parties. Most states have abortion legislation, some states have statutes regarding artificial insemination, and a few states have guidelines for genetic screening prior to the issuance of a marriage license. Physicians and their employees should be knowledgeable of their own state statutes.

The primary role of the physician is to inform patients of all aspects of genetics that may relate to their specific circumstances. It is best to allow patients to make all decisions necessary and to be only an "enabler" of the process rather than the decision-maker. Physicians should know where genetic counseling is available and what can be done for patients. University hospitals and medical clinics are a good place to begin.

In artificial insemination and/or surrogate mother programs, all agreements should be in writing. A husband's consent should be in writing if his wife is to be artificially inseminated with another man's semen. In the case of a surrogate mother, her right to the child at birth should be relinquished in a written document. The physician should certify the signatures of all involved as well as the date of insemination and file the agreement with the registrar of vital statistics or proper authority, where it shall be kept confidential and in a sealed file.[11]

Confidentiality will be the second legal implication in all matters of eugenics. Physicians and their employees must keep information in the strictest confidence at all times. It is often difficult for patients to discuss such matters freely, even with the physician. The possibility that any information might become available, although unknowingly, to a third party through an overheard telephone conversation or a mislaid medical record is intolerable both to the medical profession and to the patients. Care must be taken to preserve the dignity of all involved. Comments made by the staff need to be pertinent, informative, and helpful—not judgmental. The decision is the patients'. They alone must decide, freely and without coercion.

Any time such matters fall outside the training and education of a particular physician, referral to a place where patients can receive the help desired should be made.

REFERENCES

1. MUNSON, R: *Intervention and Reflection*. Wadsworth, 1969, p 339.
2. BEAUCHAMP, TL AND WALTERS, L: *Contemporary Issues in Bioethics*. Dickinson, Belmont, CA, 1978, pp 568-569.
3. IBID, p 570.
4. *Conception in a glass*. Time, July 31, 1978, p 59.
5. WATSON, JD: *The future of asexual reproduction. Contemporary Issues in Bioethics.* Dickinson, Belmont, CA, 1978, p 605.
6. ANDERSON, CP: *In his own words.* People, April 17, 1978, p 94.
7. OSTROM, C: *Who shall be born?* Seattle Times, March 22, 1981.
8. FRIEDMANN, T: *Prenatal diagnosis of genetic disease. Contemporary Issues in Bioethics.* Dickinson, Belmont, CA, 1978, p 575.
9. IBID, p 577.
10. BECKWITH, J: *Social and political uses of genetics in the United States: Past and present. Intervention and Reflection.* Wadsworth, 1979, p 386.
11. WASHINGTON STATE MEDICAL ASSOCIATION: *Medical-Legal Handbook.* Seattle, 1980, p 3.

DISCUSSION QUESTIONS

1. Identify one example of both negative and positive eugenics practiced in society today. Identify one in your state.

2. Should genetic screening/testing be mandatory for any disease? Support your answer.

3. Katherine is a surrogate mother for a couple living 1500 miles away. Katherine, near term of pregnancy, decides she does not want to go through with relinquishing the baby. What she does not know is that the prospective mother was killed in an auto

accident two weeks ago. Who has right to the child? How is a decision made?

4. How "normal" do we want humankind to be?

5. Describe possible problems for "test-tube babies."

6. Professor Joseph Fletcher, bioethicist, says, "It is unethical and morally wrong to deliberately or knowingly bring a diseased child into the world, or to turn a cold shoulder on prenatal tests. Never bring a baby into the world with anything more than minimally serious defects or disease." Discuss.

7. Paul Ramsey, Professor of Religion at Princeton University, says, "We cannot begin by bloodying ourselves with the killing of our own kind because they are defective in the womb, without also going to infanticide of similarly defective *born* infants." Discuss.

CHAPTER 14

ARTIFICIAL INSEMINATION

LEARNING OBJECTIVES

Upon successful completion of this chapter, you will:

1. Define AIH and AID.

2. Identify circumstances that may warrant AIH and AID.

3. List at least four problems raised by AID.

4. Describe procedures to follow in securing consent from participants of AIH and AID.

5. Recall possible sources for sperm used in artificial insemination.

6. Relate your personal feelings to the suggestions of etiquette at the end of the chapter.

DEFINITIONS

Heterologous Insemination. Injection of a donor's semen into the vagina to induce conception—AID.

Homologous Insemination. Injection of the husband's semen into the vagina to induce conception—AIH.

INTRODUCTION

The preceding chapter briefly mentioned artificial insemination as related to eugenics. The subject has complex legal and ethical ramifications for office employees and their physicians aside from its eugenics potential and should be considered separately.

As many as 25 percent of couples in the United States are unable to have children. For whatever reason, infertility seems to be on the increase. At the same time, the number of infants available for adoption has declined. One possible solution to the dilemma is artificial insemination.

Artificial insemination is not a difficult procedure. There are indications to believe that it has been practiced for thousands of years by individuals who had a strong desire to have a child. It is estimated that approximately 100,000 children are born of artificial insemination each year, and the number is growing.

Artificial insemination is considered to be AIH or AID. AIH is homologous artificial insemination by husband. AID is heterologous artificial insemination by donor. AIH might be used when a husband's sperm vitality may be too low or a woman's cervical mucus too hostile to achieve conception. Semen collected and concentrated over a period of a few days can often overcome a sperm count too low or not vital enough. AID might be used when the husband is sterile or carries serious genetic defects. It also has been used by women who want to have a child but have no desire to have sexual intercourse with a man.

Obstetricians and gynecologists are being asked about AIH and AID almost daily. Physicians in this specialty and their employees especially need to be able to discuss the topic with intelligence and understanding. Fertility clinics and specialists are often found in major cities and within a reasonable distance of women desiring AIH or AID if their personal physicians do not wish to participate. Some physicians will practice AIH but not AID, usually for legal and sometimes for ethical reasons.

LEGAL IMPLICATIONS

Physicians practicing AIH will want to exhaust all available fertility testing before recommending AIH. Upon determining to proceed with AIH, care must be taken to explain the procedure, its effectiveness, and any possible problems likely to occur. Permission to perform the procedure should be in writing, with both the husband and wife consenting. Confidentiality must be assured.

AID presents problems separate from AIH. Using the semen of a donor rather than the woman's husband raises some questions. These include (1) Does the donor have any right to the child? (2) What kind of screening should be used to determine an appropriate donor? (3) Can the physician be held liable if careful screening is not adhered to? and (4) Is an act of adultery committed?

In the past few years, more states have begun to address these questions. For the most part, however, there are few state statutes dealing with artificial insemination. Before performing AIH or AID, physicians need to be aware of their state's laws. States with no laws on the subject must rely on the dignity of physicians to act with reasonable care and to protect themselves and their patients in the process. In such states, persons seeking AID also would be wise to seek legal counsel regarding the legal protection and parentage of the offspring.

Physicians will want the signatures of both husband and wife if insemination is from a donor. One state in particular, Washington, requires these signatures and the date of insemination to be filed with the registrar of vital statistics, where the file is kept confidential and sealed similarly to adoption records. Such a procedure or one similar seems wise when considering the ramifications of records kept only by the physicians involved in such a procedure.

Counseling should be done to ascertain that both husband and wife want AID. It is more difficult for some men to accept a child of AID than an adopted child. Realistically, the opposite can be true. Some men can accept AID children born by their own wives completely as their own. That acceptance is important.

When there is no husband, physicians need only the signature of the consenting woman. The written consent of the donor is required in all cases. The donor's signature is to release all claims of paternity. The donor should not know who is receiving his semen, nor should the woman know the donor's identity. A relative also should not be considered as a donor. For the most part, selection of an appropriate donor is up to the physician. If the donor is married, consent from his wife may be a wise procedure, since her marital interests also are affected.

Some fertility clinics will have a number of donors who can be called to bring semen when asked and are usually paid a fee for their services. Other clinics may rely upon some of their employees or medical students. There are only a few sperm banks in this country, but they provide another alternative for suitable sperm.

Physicians and clinics using the services of sperm donors will want to screen carefully and meticulously. Some considerations include (1) a complete physical and psychological examination, (2) a sperm analysis, (3) a genetic history, and (4) appropriate blood tests. Some physicians prefer donors who have fathered healthy children. Careful consideration also is given to selecting a donor who has physical characteristics near those of the husband or those desired by the woman.

If "in-house" staff are used as donors, the utmost care must be taken to assure confidentiality of all involved as well as the same criteria for "on-call" donors. For example, it may be fairly easy for an intern who is a donor for a large medical setting to discover, either accidentally or purposely, the identity of a woman receiving his sperm.

Using frozen sperm for insemination may not be as successful as fresh semen, but it does make confidentiality of identity more certain if the sperm bank is some distance away. Physicians using the services of a sperm bank will want to be as careful in their selection of that bank as they would be of a laboratory to which they refer their patients.

Some physicians who perform AID will recommend the woman seek another physician if she becomes pregnant for prenatal care and delivery. This may prevent any unnecessary questions regarding paternity of the newborn and may be wise in states that have not addressed the issue.

ETHICAL IMPLICATIONS

There are some ethical questions to consider in the whole realm of artificial insemination. Does the question of sexuality being tied to the ability to procreate have validity? Society places much emphasis on fertility while adoptable children need loving parents. These children are often not infants, may be multiracial, and may have physical or psychological difficulties. Would society's emphasis be better placed on the needs of such children?

Should artificial insemination be performed on married women only? Who should be a mother? Some religious beliefs treat AID as adultery. Is the child then illegitimate?

At least one state requires that the names and dates pertaining to insemination be kept in a sealed file in the department of vital statistics. Adoption files were originally sealed, also. But these files now are becoming available to individuals wishing to know their true heritage. Is a similar possibility likely in the future for AID children?

What of states where no statutes have been enacted? Who monitors physicians practicing AID? Who assures that donors have been carefully screened? What becomes of the AID records upon the death of physicians or when their practices are closed?

Perhaps remote, but still a possibility—who has ethical responsibility to prevent the potential marriage of half-brothers and sisters through AID in the future?

Artificial insemination is a medical fact, an ethical dilemma, and a legal concern that will expand in the next few years. Most medical office employees and their physicians will deal directly with the issue during their careers. *Law and Ethics for A.I.D. and Embryo Transfer* is a book based on a symposium held at the Ciba Foundation in London December, 1972. It addresses many questions considered here and provides additional information.

Those who do not wish to be involved in AIH or AID for legal, ethical, religious, or any other reason need not be. Patient referral can be made to other physicians or clinics who do perform artificial insemination. Medical office employees who prefer not to be involved with artificial insemination should make that preference known prior to employment.

Those professionals involved in artificial insemination will want to remember that both men and women may be uncomfortable with the knowledge that several members of the medical staff know of their fertility problems and that AIH or AID is being attempted. Medical office assistants may have to ask men to manually produce their semen and to explain to women how that semen will be deposited, usually on more than one occasion, in their cervix without sexual intercourse. Treating these individuals in a professional manner, realizing that this is not a place for slapstick humor, will alleviate some of the patients' anxieties and encourage open communication.

Artificial insemination is a truly private decision and a very personal procedure. Tact and courtesy must be followed at all times, and the confidentiality and privacy of those involved carefully protected.

DISCUSSION QUESTIONS

1. Why does AID pose more of a problem, ethically and legally, than AIH?

2. A patient is in tears when she leaves the office. You ask if there is anything wrong and are told that the doctor refuses to consider AIH. You know that the woman has been trying to have a child for a long while. What can you say or do?

3. Discuss how you might handle the medical records of individuals involved in AID if the registrar of vital statistics is not interested in them.

4. Predict legal and ethical implications for the offspring of AID.

5. A couple comes into the medical office for AID. They have determined that the husband's brother should be the donor and have already made arrangements with him. What counseling would you suggest?

CHAPTER **15**

STERILIZATION

LEARNING OBJECTIVES

Upon successful completion of this chapter, you will:

1. Recall historical background of sterilization.
2. Define therapeutic, nontherapeutic, voluntary, and involuntary sterilization.
3. Explain four methods of sterilization.
4. Discuss effectiveness and reversibility of sterilization.
5. Review the legal implications of sterilization.
6. Present an ethical position *for* and *against* sterilization.
7. Describe the role of the physician and the role of the medical office employee regarding sterilization.

DEFINITIONS

Castrate. To remove the testicles or ovaries surgically.

Cauterization. Destruction of tissue by an electrical current or caustic agent.

Culdoscope. An instrument for examining the female viscera (abdominal organs) through the vagina.

Laparoscope. An instrument for examining the abdominal or peritoneal cavity that uses a fiberoptic light source.

INTRODUCTION

Sterilization is not a new issue. Babylonians castrated slaves and made them guardians of the home. Castration was a form of punishment in early Chinese civilizations. Australian aborigine tribes surgically slit along the urethra close to the testicles so that at the time of ejaculation, semen would spill out through the slit rather than be deposited in the vagina. The ovaries of women were removed in ancient Egypt.[1] This list of sterilization methods is not complete but serves as a reminder that men and women have been seeking an effective method of birth control for centuries.

Sterilization may be therapeutic or nontherapeutic, voluntary or involuntary.

Therapeutic sterilization implies the removal of all or part of the reproductive organs in order to protect the health and the life of the patient. *Nontherapeutic sterilization,* often called "convenience" sterilization, is the removal of all or part of the reproductive organs for the purpose of destroying the reproductive function. *Voluntary sterilization* is a term synonymous with nontherapeutic and convenience sterilization. *Involuntary sterilization* is compulsory sterilization of individuals for eugenic reasons.

STERILIZATION METHODS

Sterilization for women is called *tubal ligation* and involves cutting, tying, and clamping the fallopian tubes so the egg will not meet the sperm and pass into the uterus. Tubal ligations are performed abdominally or vaginally.

Sterilization within two days of childbirth involves an incision about one and one-half inches long beneath the navel and uses an instrument to pick up the tubes for cutting, tying, or clamping. This may be called *postpartum sterilization.*

Minilaparotomy, often performed for postpartum sterilization, can be done at other times as well. A small incision is made above the pubic hairline allowing the physician to insert small instruments to bring the tubes into vision. The tubes then are cut, tied, or clamped.

Laparoscopy, often called the "band-aid" surgery, involves a tiny incision in the navel to allow a laparoscope, which makes visible all parts of the abdomen, to be inserted. Carbon dioxide is injected into the abdomen to move the bowels away from the area. The most common ligation here is tubal cauterization. Laparoscopy is currently the preferred method of tubal ligation in the United States.

Culdoscopy requires an incision in the vagina, behind the cervix, for the insertion of a culdoscope and the picking up of the tubes for ligation. A local anesthetic is used because the woman is placed in a position in which she sits on her knees, hands forward, resting her chest on the table (knee-chest position). The procedure requires less than one-half hour, but is associated with considerable discomfort because of the position.

Sterilization for men is by *vasectomy*. The procedure requires a local anesthetic and a small bilateral incision into the scrotum. The vas deferens are pulled out and ligated. Follow-up of this procedure is important to assure that all of the sperm have been discharged before sterility occurs. Two consecutive sperm counts must prove negative before birth control methods should be discontinued.

EFFECTIVENESS AND REVERSIBILITY

The sterilization procedures described are nearly 100 percent effective in birth control and have little if any side effects. Sexual desires or pleasures are not affected and no hormonal body changes are made. Menstruation will continue normally.

Reversibility of the procedure is another matter. Sterilization should generally be considered permanent, even though there has been some success in reversing the procedure. Reversal is not always as simple as the operation for sterilization, and the chances of conception remain slim.

THE LAW AND STERILIZATION

Few individuals have objections to therapeutic sterilization when necessary to protect life and health. The Roman Catholic view, however, goes a step further and says that if "the operation is to prevent the inconvenience or dangers of childbearing, it is illicit."[2] The problem in therapeutic sterilization is in defining "therapeutic." Is a patient with mild diabetes less likely to receive a therapeutic sterilization than one with severe diabetes? Who makes the final decision in a therapeutic sterilization? The doctor, the patient, or the court?

Not every state has addressed the issue of sterilization. There are several states with statutes making involuntary sterilization compulsory for feeble-minded inmates of state mental institutions.[3] To date, three states, Connecticut, Kansas, and Utah, make sterilization a crime for any other reason than therapeutic or eugenic purposes. There may be reason to believe that such laws are unconstitutional.

Virginia and North Carolina have requirements for the consent of the spouse in sterilization. Georgia's General Assembly in 1966 granted physicians who perform voluntary sterilizations immunity from criminal and civil suits.[4] The absence of other laws on sterilization puts physicians and patients in a dilemma, both legally and ethically.

ETHICS AND STERILIZATION

Some patients and physicians will argue that individuals should have control over their bodies and that they alone should be able to decide whether or not sterilization should occur. There is a strong argument against sterilization for eugenic purposes, and many consider involuntary sterilization mutilation. The rights of spouses in any sterilization procedure need to be considered, since their procreation function is affected also. Arguments also have been made by the legal guardians of severely mentally retarded persons for eugenic or involuntary sterilization.

Another ethical issue to consider is whether sterilization is a valid method of contraception. Society must bear some burden for the attitudinal pressure that frowns upon large families. Some countries place severe tax penalties upon couples who have more than two children. Many countries are conscious of a severe population explosion. And partly as a result, six million vasectomies were performed in India between 1968 and 1972, and the campaign for permanent contraception continues.

Sterilization as a form of contraception also has increased in the United States. In 1969, one quarter million men had vasectomies. In 1970, it was three-quarter million—an increase of 200 percent![5] Perhaps the tide is turning in the 1980s, but the pressure still exists. And much of that pressure is brought about by the fact that the world's resources are being depleted while the population increases.

Perhaps an even more subtle ethical issue is the concern individuals have for their basic loss of personal freedoms. How much control should governments have over individuals? Will personal freedom, completely unregulated, destroy any potential for a future? Who is going to make these decisions? How will it be done?

As so often is the case, physicians and their patients will make decisions on sterilization alone, with little assistance from the law or agreed-upon ethical standards.

OFFICE PROTOCOL

It is wise, therefore, for physicians to perform sterilization procedures, for any reason, completely within state statutes and *only after* receiving written, informed consent from the individuals involved. Careful counseling should be given in all cases, especially for voluntary and/or convenience sterilization. Physicians should help patients understand that the procedure is considered permanent and will remove any possibility of having children. Care should be taken in sterilizations of young adults who are unmarried or who have no children.

Medical office employees will be in direct contact with patients seeking information or an actual sterilization. Employees will need to be knowledgeable of the sterilization procedures, their side effects, and their benefits. In many instances, employees will be asked to offer their opinions and advice. The decision, however, must be made by the patient. Employees should be good listeners and offer factual information. Employees should try to be unbiased patient advocates, confidants, and reinforcers of their physicians' regimens.

In many instances, patients will have sterilization procedures done in physicians' offices. Employees may assist both patient and physician during the procedures. If this situation produces value conflicts, employees may need to re-examine their personal feelings and their places of employment. It is important to realize that patients are making a decision that will last forever. Such decisions deserve understanding and consideration, and should be free of value judgments from employees.

Every attempt should be made to follow the best standards on informed consent and to have the signatures of all involved. Some physicians have utilized a "waiting period" after consent papers have been signed before sterilization is performed. This provides ample opportunity for those involved to reverse their decisions.

REFERENCES

1. LAUERSEN, N AND WHITNEY, S: *It's Your Body: A Woman's Guide to Gynecology.* Playboy Paperbacks, New York, 1973, pp 172-175.
2. CREIGHTON, H: *Law Every Nurse Should Know.* WB Saunders, Philadelphia, 1981, p 223.
3. LONG, R: *The Physician and the Law.* Appleton-Century-Crofts, New York, 1968, p 336.
4. CREIGHTON, p 220.
5. LAUERSEN, pp 257-258.

DISCUSSION QUESTIONS

1. Present a strong argument for sterilization; against sterilization.

2. What are the sterilization laws in your state?

3. Do you know where to refer patients for sterilization information?

4. Why is informed consent essential for a sterilization procedure?

5. Should permission of a spouse be mandatory?

6. Should sterilization be performed for eugenic purposes?

CHAPTER **16**

ABORTION

LEARNING OBJECTIVES

Upon successful completion of this chapter, you will:

1. Define abortion and miscarriage.
2. Describe the process of fetal development.
3. List five theories for when life begins.
4. Explain the methods of abortion.
5. Discuss the Supreme Court decisions on abortion from 1973 to present.
6. Analyze three major ethical issues on abortion.
7. Identify guidelines for abortion in medical offices.

DEFINITIONS

Conceptus. General term referring to any product of conception.

Eugenic Abortion. Abortion performed because the fetus is severely deformed or damaged.

Infanticide. A type of homicide consisting of killing the newborn.

Mitosis. The process by which the cell splits into two new cells, each having the same number of chromosomes as the parent cell.

Ovum. Female germ cell.

Quickening. The first perceptible movement of the fetus in the uterus.

Spermatozoon. Male germ cell.

Therapeutic Abortion. Abortion performed to preserve the life or health of the mother.

Zygote. The fertilized ovum; the cell produced by the union of gametes.

INTRODUCTION

"Whatever one's reaction to the term *abortion*, it is seldom neutral. Begin to discuss abortion and normally rational people become quite emotional and react strongly."[1] Abortion is the termination of pregnancy before the fetus is viable. Medically, the terms abortion and miscarriage both refer to the termination of pregnancy before the fetus is capable of survival outside the uterus. In general usage, abortion refers to *deliberate* termination of pregnancy, while miscarriage refers to a spontaneous or natural loss of the fetus.[2] In this chapter, abortion means the deliberate termination of pregnancy.

FETAL DEVELOPMENT

Fertilization occurs when a spermatozoon (male sperm cell) unites with an ovum (female egg) within a few hours of sexual intercourse. Normally, this takes place in the fallopian tubes, after which the fertilized ovum, now called a zygote, begins its journey to the uterus (womb). The zygote begins a process of mitosis (cell division) during the approximate 3-day journey to the uterus. Mitosis continues while the zygote floats freely in the uterus and begins to attach itself to the uterine lining. The proper term for this attached "ball of cells" is a blastocyst.

The blastocyst continues development and attachment to the uterus until firmly implanted at the end of the second week. From the second week until the end of the eighth week, the blastocyst is called an embryo. During this time organ systems begin to develop, and some features take on a human shape.

At approximately the eighth week, the embryo becomes known as a fetus and is marked by the beginning of brain activity. The term fetus is used until the time of birth, usually nine months after fertilization. The nine-month period is generally divided into three segments or *trimesters*. The first trimester is from fertilization to three months, the second trimester is from three to six months into the pregnancy, and the third trimester is from the sixth to ninth months (Table 1).

TABLE 1. Fetal Development

End of Month	Approximate Size and Weight	Representative Changes
1	3/16 inch	Eyes, nose, and ears not yet visible. Backbone and vertebral canal form. Small buds that will develop into arms and legs form. Heart forms and starts beating.
2	1 1/4 inches 1/30 ounce	Ossification begins. Limbs become distinct as arms and legs. Digits are well formed. Major blood vessels form.
3	3 inches 1 ounce	Eyes almost fully developed but eyelids still fused, and external ears are present. Appendages are fully formed. Heartbeat can be detected. Body systems continue to develop.
4	6 1/2-7 inches 4 ounces	Head large in proportion to rest of body. Face takes on human features and hair appears on head. Many bones ossified and joints begin to form.
5	10-12 inches 1/2-1 pound	Head less disproportionate to rest of body. Fine hair covers body. Rapid development of body systems.
6	11-14 inches 1 1/4-1 1/2 pounds	Head becomes even less disproportionate to rest of body. Eyelids separate and eyelashes form.
7	13-17 inches 2 1/2-3 pounds	Head and body become more proportionate. Skin wrinkled and pink. Seven-month fetus (premature) is capable of survival.
8	16 1/2-18 inches 4 1/2-5 pounds	Testes descend into scrotum. Bones of head are soft. Chances of survival are much greater at end of eighth month.
9	20 inches 7-7 1/2 pounds	Additional subcutaneous fat accumulates. Nails extend to tips of fingers.

WHEN DOES LIFE BEGIN?

Since most definitions of abortion refer to the time a fetus is viable, it is important to define viable. *Taber's Cyclopedic Medical Dictionary*[3] defines viable as being capable of living outside the uterus, usually 28 weeks or older. There is no universal consensus on the time of viability. Some sources say from 20 to 35 weeks is the time of viability. Most agree that it is rare for a fetus to survive before the twentieth week. Medical technology has made tremendous advances in keeping a premature infant alive. In underdeveloped countries, however, where there is little medical technology, the time of viability may surpass 35 weeks.

Five possible considerations of when life begins are (1) at the time of conception, (2) when the brain begins to function at 8 to 12 weeks, (3) at the time of quickening at 16 to 18 weeks, (4) at the time of viability from 20 to 35 weeks, and (5) at the time of birth.

Some religious groups, including Roman Catholics, claim that life begins at conception because the blastocyst carries the genetic code for a new human being. The theory also is seen in the Chinese and Korean cultures, which count a child as nine months or a year old at the time of birth.

Another determination for the beginning of life is at the time the brain begins to function. Proponents of this theory believe the fetus cannot be a human without a functioning brain. Since there is strong support for the idea that death occurs when the brain ceases to function, it may be logical to believe that life occurs when the brain begins to function.

Quickening has been determined by some to be the beginning of life. Aristotle believed that prior to quickening, the human fetus had only a vegetable or animal soul.[4] Another reason for this position perhaps is that women truly feel "life" at the time of quickening.

The idea that life begins when the fetus is viable or can live independently of the uterus is partly based upon the premise that if the fetus indeed can live on its own, then life has begun. More variation of time is allowed in this theory if you consider that viability may be sometime between 20 to 35 weeks.

Those who believe that life begins only at the time of actual birth believe so because now the being can be seen, can be held, and is perceived as being fully human.

METHODS OF ABORTION

The method of abortion will depend to a great extent on the stage of the pregnancy. The descriptions given are from *It's Your Body* by Lauersen and Whitney.[5]

The *"morning-after" pill,* while not a method of abortion, is the earliest intervention of possible pregnancy. The theory behind the "morning-after" pill is that high doses of estrogen over a period of days prevent the fertilized egg from implanting in the uterine lining. The pills are taken for approximately five days and must be started within 72 hours of unprotected intercourse. The "morning-after" pills are often used in the case of rape or incest.

The safest and quickest method of abortion, if a pregnancy test is positive and it is less than seven weeks from the last menstruation, is called vacuum aspiration or *miniabortion.* In this procedure a tube with a suction device is inserted through the cervix into the uterus. (Dilation is usually unnecessary.) Within one or two minutes, the lining on the uterine wall and the conceptus are suctioned out. Cramping, nausea, and faintness may be experienced by a woman undergoing this procedure. It is commonly performed in the medical office.

If pregnancy is terminated between the seventh and twelfth weeks, a *suction abortion or curettage* is performed. The procedure is similar to the miniabortion. In the medical office or clinic, a local anesthetic is given and the cervix is dilated to permit suction and scraping of the uterine lining. In a hospital, a general anesthetic is used. Cramping, nausea, and vomiting usually follow the procedure. The patient can go home about two hours afterward.

The preceding methods of abortion occur in the first trimester—up to 12 weeks of pregnancy. The period of 12 to 16 weeks affords few safe methods of abortion, because the fetus is too large for a suction abortion and there is insufficient amniotic fluid for a saline injection. During this time, two methods are the use of repeated *vaginal or intramuscular administrations of prostaglandins,* which encourage expulsion of the conceptus within 10 to 15 hours. The methods are relatively new and lengthy procedures that require close observation. Research is likely soon to produce other prostaglandin methods for the 12- to 16-week period of gestation that will be less complex and easier to administer.

The *saline injection* is performed during the sixteenth to twenty-fourth weeks of gestation. The procedure involves withdrawing between 50 to 200 cc of amniotic fluid through a needle and syringe. Approximately 200 cc of saline solution is then slowly injected into the remaining amniotic fluid. This procedure brings about normal labor and delivery of the fetus within 18 to 20 hours. The same procedure is followed to instill prostaglandin into the amniotic sac except only a small amount of amniotic fluid is removed. The results are the same. These procedures can be performed only in a hospital and require 1 1/2 to 3 days' stay.

In a very few cases a *hysterotomy* or *minicaesarean section* is performed to remove the fetus surgically. This is considered major surgery, requiring six to eight days' hospitalization and a longer period of recuperation than any other method. It is usually performed only in the case of uterine abnormalities.

Generally, the later an abortion of any type is performed, the greater the risk. Psychological and physiological difficulties can and may accompany any method of abortion. When pregnancy is to be terminated, for any reason, only qualified physicians and appropriate facilities should be used. Women are advised to seek professional help as soon as possible for their own safety and well-being.

ABORTION AND THE LAW

In 1800 no abortion laws existed in the United States. When a woman wanted an abortion, she received it. By 1900 nearly every state had laws prohibiting abortion and treating it as a criminal offense. Eighty years later, federal and state abortion laws still exist, but tend to allow more freedom than those in the early 1900s.

One of the monumental decisions affecting a change of all abortion laws was the 1973 United States Supreme Court *Roe v. Wade* decision. Jane Roe, a pseudonym, was a single, pregnant woman, who took action against Henry Wade, the District Attorney of Dallas County, in 1970. Roe pleaded the Fourteenth Amendment and her "right to privacy," claiming the Texas anti-abortion statute unconstitutional.[6] As a result, three years later the Supreme Court held that during the first trimester, pregnant women have a constitutional right to abortions and the state has no vested interest at that time. During the second trimester the state may regulate abortion,[7] and insist upon reasonable standards of medical practice if an abortion is to be performed. During the third trimester the state may override pregnant women's rights to abortions, and the state could "proscribe abortion except when necessary to preserve the health or life of the mother."[8]

Although this court decision did "favor" Roe, many unanswered questions resulted. For example, when is the fetus viable? Is the fetus "property" of the bearer? Does the woman alone have the right or do spouses/parents have rights? Can state and/or federal funding be required for abortions? Virtually every state statute on abortion was invalidated, either partly or totally, by the Roe Supreme Court decision. The public responded to their legislators, who, in turn, reacted through legislation. Some state laws were thus more restrictive than the Supreme Court decisions. Some state statutes set facility requirements where abortions were to be performed, others addressed filing of detailed reports on abortions performed, what consultation needs to be done prior to an abortion, and other such requirements.[9]

Another United States Supreme Court decision in 1976 changed state abortion statutes. The court ruled on constitutional grounds, that spouse and parent consent is not necessary for an abortion of a wife or a daughter. Currently courts tend not to differentiate between minor and adult pregnant women.[10] Absolute parental consent may force pregnant minors to seek criminal or self-induced abortions. A 1978 United States Supreme Court decision held that a state may not constitutionally legislate a blanket, unreviewable power of parents to veto their daughter's abortion.

In the 1977 *Doe v. Bolton* case, the Supreme Court struck down four preabortion procedural requirements: (1) residency, (2) performance of the abortion in a hospital accredited by the JCAH, (3) approval by a committee of the hospital's medical staff, and (4) consultations.[11] It also had a "conscience clause" stating that physicians and medical employees could refuse to participate in abortions without being discriminated against.

In June 1977, three related cases, *Real v. Doe, Maher v. Doe* and *Poelker v. Doe*, resulted in Supreme Court decisions also affecting abortion laws. The ruling stated "that the states have neither a constitutional nor a statutory obligation under Medicaid to provide nontherapeutic abortions for indigent women or access to public facilities for the performance of such abortions."[12] Recently, the court held that federal funding of abortion has been available only when the mother's life is endangered or in cases of incest or rape. Although states may use their own revenues for nontherapeutic abortions, six states follow the federal criteria;* 22 jurisdictions have no restrictions;† 15 states follow the federal criteria but also permit abortion when severe damage to physical health would result;†† and seven states provide funding only when the life of the mother is endangered.¶[13]

Legal challenges are currently in the process and more Supreme Court decisions are expected. The majority of abortion questions arise over the Fourteenth Amendment and the equal protection clause. Every citizen of the United States has "equal protection of the law," and shall not be discriminated against. This includes abortion. The states, then, are testing the courts both on "strict scrutiny" and "rational basis." For example, is it discriminatory for a woman who has money and/or insurance coverage to receive an abortion, and a woman who is poor and relies on welfare to be denied an abortion? Will this withstand the "strict scrutiny" of the court on discrimination? Is there a "rational basis" for discrimination in the case of an unmarried woman versus a married woman seeking abortions? Can states require married women to obtain their husbands' consent?

The abortion issue and its laws are in a state of flux. Radical changes have occurred in the last one hundred years. Who could predict what the next one hundred years will bring? The political climate, moral attitudes, advances in medical technology, and the impact of current abortion laws will influence the future of abortion.

ETHICS AND ABORTION

Three major ethical issues surface in a discussion on abortion. It seems invalid to consider these issues separately. To do so is being neither honest nor realistic. The issues are:

1. Are there any reasons to justify abortions?
2. Are current laws regarding abortions consistent, fair, and just?
3. Are abortions an appropriate method of birth control?

---

*Iowa, Kansas, Massachusetts, Missouri, New Mexico, Utah.

†Alaska, California, Colorado, Connecticut, Georgia, Hawaii, Illinois, Louisiana, Maryland, Michigan, Minnesota, New Jersey, New York, North Carolina, Ohio, Oregon, Pennsylvania, Virginia, Washington, West Virginia, Wisconsin, District of Columbia.

††Alabama, Arkansas, Delaware, Florida, Idaho, Maine, Mississippi, Montana, Nevada, New Hampshire, Oklahoma, South Carolina, Tennessee, Texas, Vermont.

¶Indiana, Kentucky, Nebraska, North Dakota, Rhode Island, South Dakota, Wyoming.

1. "ARE THERE ANY REASONS TO JUSTIFY ABORTIONS?"

An immediate answer may be "Yes," "No," "In at least two situations," or "It depends upon the circumstances."

To answer "Yes" with no restrictions implies that abortions should be performed upon demand and at any time during the pregnancy and still be safe. The viability of the fetus or the circumstances are not issues to consider. The issue is a woman's right to make a decision on whether, if, or when an abortion is to be performed. The pregnant woman's right is higher than any other. The issue is one of freedom and human rights. Proponents of this theory may be labeled *pro-abortion*.

To answer "No" without any other consideration is to believe that abortion for any reason is murder. The consideration here is that the fetus is innocent, weak, and helpless and its right to life should be protected at all costs. These individuals often believe that to allow abortion is to also condone infanticide. The rights of the fetus and newborn are paramount to the rights of any others. Proponents of this theory may be called *pro-life*.

To answer "In at least two situations" or "It depends upon the circumstances" is a stand somewhere in the middle of pro-abortion and pro-life. These individuals are often labeled *pro-choice*. There are the advocates who believe that abortion is permissible to save the life of the mother. This is one situation that receives quite a bit of support from *pro-choice* individuals. The second situation making abortion permissible and receiving support is in the case of rape or incest. If the response to the question is, "It depends upon the circumstances," then each set of circumstances will determine whether an abortion is performed or the fetus is allowed to survive. This premise considers the rights of both mother and fetus and the rights of any others who may be involved. Most likely, pro-choice individuals also consider the question of when life begins.

One may expect that the church offers a solution to the question of when life begins. In discussing ethical questions, actions of the church are often considered. But there is no consensus or agreement here which settles the issue. There are a few religious groups who propose that abortions be performed only when necessary to save the mother's life. Some religious groups determine a time or establish viability of the fetus for performing abortions. All make an attempt to understand the pain and trauma associated with any decision on abortion.

2. "ARE CURRENT LAWS REGARDING ABORTIONS CONSISTENT, FAIR, AND JUST?"

This second ethical question may be somewhat easier to answer than the first. However, there is no general agreement on a response here either.

As was discussed earlier, laws were fairly consistent in the early 1900s. Abortions were illegal. The issue came into full public view in 1973 with the

Roe v. Wade Supreme Court decision. Statutes then changed, and abortion became legal.

These statutes are inconsistent, however. The Supreme Court's intentionally vague ruling has left the states to interpret and regulate abortions. Much variation remains. There is little agreement on the viability of the fetus or what regulations, if any, are established for physicians and facilities. Therefore, abortions may be completely legal in one state, but not in another.

The consideration of how abortions are to be funded is even more complex. The 1977 Supreme Court ruling that said states were not required to fund abortions for the indigent woman raises the question of fairness and justice in following the law. Essentially, this ruling has the force of denying an abortion to a woman unable to pay. The right to choose becomes hinged upon the ability to pay. This, in effect, denies personal freedom in a free society that has guaranteed it under the Fourteenth Amendment. The other side of the coin means that strong opponents of abortion will pay through their taxes in Medicaid funding for those who choose abortion. Persons who object on this basis also must weigh the costs of a funded abortion against the pregnancy, delivery, and welfare costs of the mother and child.

Statistics become outdated quickly, but a comparison study made in 1980 in the state of Washington is revealing. The cost to the state for 5,307 legal abortions of low-income women was $1,126,000. If the same women had given birth and, of necessity, enrolled on welfare, the cost to the state in *one year for each pregnancy* would have been $30,881,433.[14] Another financial consideration to be faced is the care, support, and institutionalizing of severely deformed infants born if eugenic abortions are not allowed. One cannot hold that abortions are morally wrong and, therefore, should not be funded, without being an advocate of health facilities that provide care for babies who require institutionalization.

3. "ARE ABORTIONS AN APPROPRIATE METHOD OF BIRTH CONTROL?"

The third ethical issue is the most recent issue and has the least information available for discussion. The two highest incidences of "abortions upon demand" come from individuals who do not practice birth control because it is not available to them and/or because it is not convenient. These groups are from the ages of 15 to 19 and from 20 to 24.

Without debating contraception, for one reason or another, contraception was not practiced and the pregnant women sought an abortion. This is further complicated by data indicating some of the same women return a second or third time for abortions.

Is something amiss in the moral standards of our society that may cause or force a teen-ager to seek an abortion because she felt too guilty or ashamed to practice contraception? Perhaps the problem is one of nonexistent or outdated sex education in a society which has become more open and accepting.

Perhaps the problem has developed because easily accessible abortions have encouraged sex without responsibility. Is information about abortions more readily available than information on contraception? Is sex education, whether in the home or school, adequate? Are parents intentional and realistic about teaching morals? Bringing a new human being into the world is a privilege and a responsibility, and it should not be left to accident as a result of exploitation, fear, or ignorance.

There is no quick, easy response to this dilemma, and the problem is growing. Repeated abortions may affect future pregnancies. The psychological impact of convenience abortions is not yet fully understood. As a society, we have not yet felt the full force of the medical or ethical ramifications of this issue.

MEDICAL OFFICE PROTOCOL

Physicians and employees must understand their own feelings on abortion. Those feelings should be based on medical fact. Their personal understanding of abortion will enable them to make a decision prior to their actual involvement. Legally, employees and physicians cannot be forced to participate in abortions against their wishes. The right to refuse, however, does not authorize the right to judge.

Physicians and employees who participate in abortions are wise to adhere to the following:

1. Participate only within the law.
2. Provide medical knowledge to patients on the stages of pregnancy, viability of the fetus, and methods of abortion.
3. Obtain written, informed consent.
4. Provide counseling as indicated by the situation.
5. Refer as necessary.
6. Keep records confidential.
7. Seek legal counsel when indicated.
8. Be understanding and compassionate.

REFERENCES

1.   HEMELT, MD AND MACKERT, ME: *Dynamics of Law in Nursing and Health Care.* Reston, Boston, 1978, p 68.
2.   MILLER, BF AND KEANE, CB: *Encyclopedia and Dictionary of Medicine and Nursing.* WB Saunders, Philadelphia, 1972, p 2.
3.   *Taber's Cyclopedic Medical Dictionary,* ed 14. FA Davis, Philadelphia, 1981, p 1554.
4.   THOMPSON, JB AND THOMPSON, HO: *Ethics in Nursing.* Macmillan, New York, 1981, p 75.

5. LAUERSEN, N AND WHITNEY, S: *It's Your Body: A Woman's Guide to Gynecology.* Playboy Paperbacks, 1977, pp 226-278.

6. MOHR, JC: *Abortion in America.* Oxford University Press, New York, 1978, p 247.

7. HEMELT, p 70.

8. MOHR, p 249.

9. STREIFF, CJ AND THE HEALTH LAW CENTER (eds): *Nursing and the Law,* ed 2. Aspen Systems Corporation, Rockville, MD, 1978, p 108.

10. IBID, p 107.

11. GALVIN, JH AND MENDELSOHN, E: *The legal status of women.* Reprinted from *The Book of the States,* 1980-1981, published by The Council of State Governments, p 39.

12. IBID.

13. IBID., p 43.

14. ASSISTANT SECRETARY OF MANAGEMENT SERVICES: *State of Washington Vital Statistics.* Department of Social and Health Services, Washington, 1980.

DISCUSSION QUESTIONS

1. In your own words, describe the process occurring in fetal development.

2. Prepare a two-minute speech for laypersons on the methods of abortion.

3. As an anti-abortionist, how would you respond to these problems:
   (a) pregnancies and resultant births from rape or incest
   (b) unwanted children
   (c) infants with severe birth defects.

4. As a pro-lifer, how would you respond to these problems:
   (a) abortion as contraception
   (b) a live aborted fetus
   (c) the right to life versus the right to freedom.

5. Where might you refer a patient for abortion counseling in your community?

6. Outline the Supreme Court rulings in the 1970s and 1980s on abortion.

7. Under what conditions is an abortion legal in your state?

8. Your physician begins to perform miniabortions and you are not sure you can participate. What will you do?

CHAPTER 17

PROLONGING LIFE/ POSTPONING DEATH BY ARTIFICIAL MEANS

LEARNING OBJECTIVES

Upon successful completion of this chapter, you will:

1. Recall examples of prolonging life and postponing death.

2. Discuss ethical considerations in prolonging life and postponing death.

3. Describe three court cases and their impact on postponing death.

4. Explain the use of an ethics committee.

5. Identify possible participants on an ethics committee.

6. Define the role of the health professional in dealing with patients and families in prolonging life/postponing death by artificial means.

DEFINITIONS

"Code Red." Medical slang indicating a life-death emergency.

Sapience. Wisdom, sageness.

INTRODUCTION

At some time in our lives, each of us will face the issue of prolonging life or postponing death by artificial means. Whether to prolong life is seldom a serious problem. The decision is made with little forethought or question. When the physician tells your wife that a cardiac pacemaker is necessary to regulate the heart beat, the general response is, "When can it be done?"

Postponing death by artificial means, however, usually involves some thought and consideration. When your wife is hospitalized with a heart condition that is rapidly deteriorating and little can be done, the question of postponing death is much more serious. When the heart monitor indicates with a buzz and a continuous monotone sound that the heart has ceased to beat, somewhere, someone is going to ask, "Do we resuscitate?"

PROLONGING LIFE BY ARTIFICIAL MEANS

Prolonging life is seldom a topic for discussion in legal or ethical circles because postponing death by artificial means is a much greater concern. Unless the quality of life and how it is preserved are understood, the question of when to postpone death is moot. To realize that life is finite, but that each of us has a right to live life to the fullest of our abilities, is an important concept to health care providers.

Most of our lives we prolong or shorten life. A well-balanced diet, appropriate weight, proper exercise, and adequate rest all can be seen as ways of prolonging life. On the other hand, smoking two packages of cigarettes a day, excessive use of alcohol, obesity, and driving recklessly may all be interpreted as shortening life. Some might say that is hastening death. It is all a matter of your value on life. Yet, such choices are often made with little thought that they may prolong life or hasten death.

Examples of prolonging life by artificial means include the use of insulin for a diabetic patient, a cardiac pacemaker for a weak heart, renal dialysis for kidney failure, and bypass surgery for clogged arteries. Generally, these are thought of as "improving" the quality of life. These choices usually are made with the knowledge that life will be prolonged because of the action taken. The finiteness of life is made known by the circumstances. Our mortality becomes real.

Few for whom life has meaning would turn their backs on the technology that has added years of life for so many. Such advances in medicine are heralded by the populace. But this technology has heightened our awareness of death at the same time it increases our life-span.

POSTPONING DEATH BY ARTIFICIAL MEANS

Every day medical personnel are confronted with whether or not to postpone death by artificial means. Should patients be allowed to die? Where is the fine line between helping to live and allowing to die? When are decisions made to use extraordinary means? What is extraordinary? What are the legal implications if physicians withhold or withdraw treatment? What is the significance of a nurse or assistant "going against" either the physician's orders or the patient's wishes? Is there a difference between human need and human right?

Examples of postponing death by artificial means may include administering ordinary or heroic CPR (cardiopulmonary resuscitation), keeping the patient on a respirator, administering medications such as antibiotics or chemotherapy when death is considered imminent, or performing a tracheotomy "as a last resort."

Each of us will die. From the moment we are born, we begin to die. Each day of life moves us closer to our death. Some of us will die suddenly and peacefully in our sleep. Some of us will die suddenly as a result of an accident. Some of us will die slowly and gradually with our bodies deteriorating and our organs ceasing to function. Some of us will die with little or no pain or discomfort. Some of us will die following great pain and discomfort. Most of us want to live, but when faced with death, desire to go quickly, painlessly and with dignity. But not all of us will be so fortunate.

Consider the following example from Dr. Donald M. Hayes[1] in *Between Doctor and Patient:*

Mr. Baker had terminal kidney failure and was comatose. Several tubes came from various places in his body. He was receiving both blood and glucose into his veins. One night he went into cardiac arrest. A team of nurses and physicians responded with a "Code Red" and worked vigorously to resuscitate. The attempt was futile and Mr. Baker died.

The memory of Mr. Baker's death was lasting to Mr. Rogers, the recently admitted patient in the same room. He said to his physician, "Please don't ever let that happen to me. I've tried all my life to live like a man; I want to die like one." Mr. Rogers underwent surgery that revealed inoperable, widespread cancer. He did not respond well, and a few days later was found with a tube in his stomach, a catheter in his bladder, a tube through his nose, and intravenous tubes into both arms. When he suffered respiratory failure, a tracheotomy was performed to save his life. He was given a slate to write on, since a tracheotomy precludes speech. Later one evening, before he managed to switch off his respirator so that he might die peacefully, he wrote on the slate, "Doctor, remember; the enemy is not death. The enemy is inhumanity."

ETHICAL CONSIDERATIONS

The ethical dilemma of prolonging life or postponing death is endless. There are many factors to consider. They include: Who makes the decision? Whose right is paramount—the patient's or the health care providers'? Do circumstances influence decisions? If so, what are they? What is ordinary and extraordinary treatment? Should resuscitation be started? Should treatment be withheld?

Who makes the decision is not easy to determine. Patients like to believe they do. Many times physicians alone decide. The burden of such decisions is heavy. If a decision is required in an instant on a life/death matter, those in closest physical proximity to the patient will decide. An emergency medical technician (EMT) will take measures instantly to save a life at the scene of an accident. Cardiac arrest on a deserted street may end in death because the only person nearby has no knowledge of what to do.

In health care facilities, the law may determine who decides. A main function of such facilities is to preserve life. If there is any question, consideration is given to the wishes of the patient, the wishes of the family, the recommendations of the physician, and perhaps the recommendations of a professional team of individuals whose purpose is to make a decision.

The problem arises over whose right is paramount in a decision. There are times when it is obvious. If a patient is unable to decide, for whatever reason, others are considered. Family will have an influence. The case of Karen Ann Quinlan demonstrated that the influence of family is not without difficulty, however. The same is often true of a patient's wishes. Even if patients are able to express their wishes to physicians and health care providers, circumstances may override them.

There are circumstances that influence decisions. Age is a factor. Resuscitation may be started on a 16-year-old, and not for an 89-year-old. Cost is a factor. Triple cardiac bypass surgery may be performed for someone of substantial means more readily than for the indigent derelict. Health is a factor. A pacemaker may be inserted for the elderly patient whose general health is good. It may be avoided if health is poor and there are other severe physical difficulties. The availability of resources is a factor. Where there is only one kidney, and four needy persons, three will do without.

We could go on. Other factors may be religion, personal philosophy of life, the amount of pain one can endure, whether a patient is comatose, and the patient's feelings on a good life versus a good death. All these factors are relative. Some are old at 45, others are young at 90. Some can endure great pain, others have a low threshold of pain. What is poor health to one person may be seen as good health to another. The relativity of the factors complicates the decision and mandates that each decision be considered individually on its own merits.

Ordinary and extraordinary treatment also is relative. You may think a heart transplant is a senseless waste of resources and money until your only chance for survival is to have one. Dialysis, once considered to be extraordinary treatment, is more commonplace today.

Understanding the relativity of circumstances that influence ethical decisions on this matter makes it difficult to respond to the questions, "Should resuscitation be started?" "Should treatment be withheld?"

Erich Fromm, a world-famous psychoanalyst, has said, "I think there is no such thing as medical ethics. There are only universal human ethics applied to specific human situations." Elisabeth Kübler-Ross[2] advises that we all have to put ourselves into the situation of the patient *first* when making a decision. Health care professionals who see death as a final stage of life rather than an evil to be thwarted at any cost will have an easier time being objective in their decision-making.

LEGAL IMPLICATIONS

Most legal rulings on prolonging life/postponing death center around "Who decides?" Prolonging life by artificial means usually poses few legal problems. Federal laws state that kidney patients have the right to the use of kidney dialysis machines as well as the necessary funding. Many individuals also have found that insulin injections are relatively inexpensive and easy to self-administer. Even insulin pumps, although somewhat inconvenient, are within economic reach, but there is no legal problem presented by their use.

Postponing death by artificial means, however, is a complex legal controversy. Perhaps the best known litigation concerns Karen Ann Quinlan. She is a New Jersey woman who, at age 21, was taken to the hospital in a comatose state by friends after a birthday party. No one is sure exactly what happened to Karen on Tuesday, April 14, 1975, but the world soon began to follow her life closely. Karen's condition deteriorated, and on July 31, her parents gave her physicians permission to take Karen off the respirator and signed a letter to that effect. The physicians morally disagreed, and told the parents. On September 12, the attorney for Joseph Quinlan, Karen's father, filed a plea with the Superior Court on three constitutional grounds: (1) the right to privacy, (2) religious freedom, and (3) cruel and unusual punishment.

Judge Robert Muir ruled against Joseph Quinlan, who then appealed the decision to the New Jersey Supreme Court. The Supreme Court decision was in Joseph Quinlan's favor and set aside any criminal liability for removing the respirator. It further recommended that Karen's physicians consult the hospital Ethics Committee to concur with their prognosis of Karen. Weeks later Karen was "weaned" from the machine. She is now without any machines and is alive seven years later.[3]

Other court decisions addressing who decides are the Saikewicz and Brother Fox cases. Saikewicz was a 76-year-old mentally retarded man with terminal cancer. Chemotherapy would prolong his life only a short time and his legal guardian thought it too cruel a burden. However, Saikewicz's close friends, with whom he spent most of his life, wanted the treatment. The court decided in favor of the guardian. Chemotherapy was not given. The High Court affirmed, decreeing that the decision belonged in court.[4]

In Brother Fox's case, the courts decided in favor of the Brother's religious superior. Brother Fox was an active 85-year-old priest who suffered a cardiac arrest during a surgical hernia repair. Brother Fox sustained substantial brain damage, was comatose, and showed "little sign of ever regaining a state of sapience or consciousness." His superior obtained two neurological consultations, discussed the situation with the family, and asked the hospital to discontinue the respirator. The lower court favored the Father, but the decision was appealed. Brother Fox died before the final ruling was made.[5]

Eight states have passed "right to die" laws in response to these cases. They include California, Oregon, New Mexico, Nevada, Arkansas, North Carolina, Idaho, and Texas. In 1979, bills dealing with the problems created by technology that prolongs the dying process where there is no hope of recovery were before legislatures in Colorado, Georgia, Kansas, Maryland, Massachusetts, Michigan, Mississippi, Missouri, New Jersey, New York, Oklahoma, South Carolina, and Washington.[6]

Many physicians think the courts have done a poor job in their decision-making regarding prolonging life/postponing death. They feel the courts are less qualified than physicians. Consequently, physicians are attempting to solve disputes through ethics committees. Elisabeth Kübler-Ross states the ideal committee includes the physician who treats the patient, any consultants, a member of the clergy, a social worker, a nurse, and a consulting psychiatrist. The committee needs to understand the family's needs as well as the patient's. Once the committee makes a decision, it informs the patient and family without asking their opinion. Thus, if the patient dies, the committee "takes" the guilt, not the family.

No one should expect bioethicists, any more than courts of law, to produce neat guidelines or ready formulas for a question so fundamentally subjective as when it may be more humane to allow a person to die or live. Doctors and nurses and patients' families will still have to confront awful choices armed with little more than their consciences, their humanity, and their moral courage.

ROLE OF HEALTH PROFESSIONALS

Any decisions medical office employees will make regarding prolonging life/postponing death by artificial means will be only in personal relationships with their families and friends rather than in any professional capacity. They may, however, often be involved in conversations with patients or their families who are struggling with the question. They also may be sounding boards to their physicians involved in the decision-making process.

As has been said before, office employees and physicians must be understanding and compassionate. Every attempt must be made to know the feelings of patients and their families. It is important that families be allowed to express any guilt they may feel in making decisions. A clear picture of the circumstances, explained by the physician in words patients can comprehend, will alleviate much of that problem. Patients who have strong feelings about having their death postponed should be encouraged to make their wishes known.

When physicians or employees are confronted with situations or questions they cannot handle, consultations and referrals should be sought. Attorneys may be called and medical societies may offer assistance. Hospital ethics committees may be valuable. Hospital chaplains, staff psychiatrists, and social workers are especially trained to help others with these personal and professional issues. Decisions of the kind discussed in this chapter weigh heavily on the minds of those involved. That weight should not be allowed to become too great.

REFERENCES

1. HAYES, DM: *Between Doctor and Patient.* Judson, Valley Forge, 1977, pp 9-11.

2. KÜBLER-ROSS, E: *Questions and Answers on Death and Dying.* Macmillan, New York, 1974, p 5.

3. MUNSON, R: *Intervention and Reflection.* Wadsworth, Belmont, CA, 1979, pp 135-138.

4. CLARK, M., GOSNELL, M and SHAPIRO, D: *When doctors play god. Newsweek,* August 31, 1981, pp 51-52.

5. REED, EA; *The case of Brother Fox. Legal Aspects of Medical Practice,* Vol 9, No 5 (May 1981), p 1.

6. CREIGHTON: *Law Every Nurse Should Know.* WB Saunders, Philadelphia, 1981, p 224.

7. KÜBLER-ROSS, pp 78-79.

8. CLARK, p 54.

DISCUSSION QUESTIONS

1. Refer to the example of Baker and Rogers at the beginning of the chapter. What would you do if you were the physician? What would you do if you were a loved one? Would your actions cause any difficulties? If so, describe.

2. If you knew that you would be put in the same situation as Karen Ann Quinlan, what would you wish?

3. Describe circumstances in which a patient is unable to make a decision on prolonging life/postponing death.

continues on next page

4. As a social worker on an ethics committee, what would you need to know to make a decision?

5. A family member comes to the medical office. She is angered because the hospital "won't stop their endless testing" and "keeps trying the impossible with my husband." What is your response?

6. A surgical patient with a guarded prognosis initiates a conversation with the physician, "If I'm not going to make it, don't let me suffer." How can the physician respond?

CHAPTER 18

EUTHANASIA

LEARNING OBJECTIVES

Upon successful completion of this chapter, you will:

1. Define euthanasia.
2. Compare passive euthanasia and active euthanasia.
3. Give at least two examples each of passive and active euthanasia.
4. Describe possible legal implications of euthanasia.
5. Discuss ethical implications of euthanasia.
6. Define the role of health professionals in euthanasia.

INTRODUCTION

Euthanasia literally means "good death." It may be defined further as a painless and easy death. But the term also can refer to the act of causing death or the painless termination of human life to end physical suffering. This latter definition is often referred to as "mercy killing."

For the purposes of this book, euthanasia will be identified as either "passive" or "active." Passive euthanasia is the withholding of treatment to allow the patient to die as soon as possible. Active euthanasia is an intentional and direct action that will kill the patient.

PASSIVE EUTHANASIA

Examples of passive euthanasia include withholding antibiotics from a terminal cancer patient who is near death and suffering from pneumonia. Or consider the patient who has terminal cancer that has metastasized and spread through the body. The patient is heavily sedated and barely alive. When the patient suddenly develops cardiac arrest, the attending physician does not start cardiac massage or try to shock the heart back to beating. The patient dies. Another patient is being kept alive by a respirator. Only the heart monitor confirms any form of life—the heart beat. But there is no recognition, no awareness, no sense of living. After a careful assessment of the situation and a discussion with family members, the medical staff decides to turn off the equipment. Life support ceases. In a matter of minutes the heart monitor indicates a steady hum rather than a heart beat. Death has occurred.

Some health professionals will deny it, but passive euthanasia is and has been an accepted medical practice for patients in their last hours of life. Many physicians have refrained from employing *extraordinary* means of preserving life while doing whatever possible by *ordinary* means to keep life going. This is a form of passive euthanasia.

ACTIVE EUTHANASIA

Active euthanasia has less support, of course, than passive euthanasia because of the stigma that the act may be considered equal to murder. Examples include leaving the patient an overdose of a narcotic or sedative that will assist dying persons to take their own lives. In this form of active euthanasia, the physician does not have a direct role in the act. Another example is the patient who requests that the physician administer an injection or prescribe a lethal dose from which the patient will not recover. Still another form of active euthanasia involves a decision made by someone rather than the patient for ending the patient's life.

Active euthanasia is a deed considered murder in most respects and bears with it severe penalty. While active euthanasia is regularly practiced with animals, it is not accepted practice with human beings.

To this point, euthanasia has been considered a dilemma for the health professional, but that is not necessarily the case. There are many circumstances of family members, spouses, loved ones, close friends, who committed either passive or active euthanasia in the case of a person near death. Many of the situations of active euthanasia are so heart-rending that jurors have great difficulties in calling it murder. Perhaps the reason is that none of us is quite certain how we will react in a given situation until that moment occurs. We certainly *think* we know how we will act, but we really do not *know*.

LEGAL IMPLICATIONS

Legal implications of euthanasia are not easily defined. There are essentially no statutes on the subject other than those that make active euthanasia murder. There are, however, some states, that because of their writing in their "Living Will" statutes, have opened the doors to legal active euthanasia. (Living Wills are discussed in Chapter 19).

The Idaho law states that "euthanasia could be actively administered to one who signed the document and who has . . . "[1] and goes on to identify conditions that may warrant the act. Some state statutes specifically state that active euthanasia is not permitted. Other state statutes are so vague in their writing as to make even the interpretation of passive euthanasia fraught with difficulties.

Some questions to ponder on the subject include the following: If euthanasia were legalized, would there be a "conscience clause" similar to abortion legislation? Who would be allowed to commit euthanasia? Is it possible that we might have "Euthanasia Planning Clinics" much like we have Planned Parenthood Clinics? If there was uniform euthanasia legislation, how would it be administered? What penalty would result if a patient's wishes on euthanasia were not followed? If physicians could commit active euthanasia, would any patients trust them?

One thing is certain, legalization of euthanasia could be as controversial, contradictory, and confusing as the legalization of abortion has been in the United States.

ETHICAL IMPLICATIONS

There is no one ethical guideline adequate for a statement on euthanasia— active or passive. One ethical view is that voluntary euthanasia is suicide and that both passive and active euthanasia are murder either because of the act of omission or comission. Tied closely with this view is the thought that only God has the right to decide at what moment a person should die, and that euthanasia violates the biblical command, "Thou shall not kill." Some religious sects believe that suffering is a part of a divine plan for every person.

A careful examination of these attitudes prompts such thoughts as "God wants each of us to live, but when it comes time to die, cannot possibly wish a bad death for anyone." Often the proponents for "Thou shall not kill" have no difficulty with killing on the battlefield and will go to great lengths to justify war biblically.

There is also the possibility that patients pronounced incurable may actually recover. That would be impossible if euthanasia had already been committed. It is conceivable that patients suffering greatly may request euthanasia on the spur of the moment with little thought of ramifications.

This, too, is impossible if euthanasia is illegal. There are those who believe that legal euthanasia would weaken the moral fiber of a country and may lead to euthanasia for only eugenic reasons. If we can commit active euthanasia for one individual to prevent further suffering, why not for severely deformed infants who have no possibility of a "normal" life?

While physicians are not demanding active euthanasia legislation of their state legislators, there are few who have not seen cases where they would have supported active euthanasia. Consider the circumstances of an infant born with severe congenital defects and intestinal obstructions requiring surgery. The medical staff and parents may decide not to operate and let the infant die. Allowing this to occur is not easy. It means watching a tiny infant gradually dehydrate and suffer from infection over a period of perhaps days. The ordeal can be terrible. While parents are protected from this experience, the medical staff is not. Many physicians and health professionals will ask, "Would it not be more merciful to inject the infant with a lethal dose of medication that would cause death to come quickly and painlessly and prevent the suffering caused by the passive euthanasia?"

In the above circumstances, some health professionals would prefer that the infant be allowed to live and that everything possible be done to enable that. Persons with this attitude, however, also must be willing to encourage state and Federal governments to provide the care that may be necessary for such infants if parents are unable.

Perhaps even more personal and difficult questions are How do I want to die? What kind of life-saving measures would I want? Do I prefer active euthanasia to passive? Can I stand to suffer? Do I have any control over my own death? Do I have a right to die as I choose? What would I want health professionals to do for me?

THE ROLE OF HEALTH PROFESSIONALS

Medical office employees will not make decisions of euthanasia in any professional capacity. Their physician employers, however, will. Perhaps the only guideline that can be offered here to the physicians is to use your best judgment, and perform only what can be allowed in your own good conscience. While some argue that we should not have to depend upon the physician's conscience, there may be little else to use as a guide. Certainly the law should be followed, religious practices considered, and the patient's rights protected when possible. But no clearly established guideline is available.

Patients who willingly and openly discuss their beliefs and wishes concerning their own death should be encouraged to complete a Living Will for their family and physician. Legal counsel should be recommended to persons if it seems appropriate. Patients should not be made to feel ashamed or guilty because of their feelings about euthanasia, no matter how much they differ from yours.

REFERENCES

1.   *Death with dignity. The International Journal of Medicine and Law* 1:2, Haifa, Israel, 1979, p 184.

DISCUSSION QUESTIONS

1. Under what circumstances might physicians and family members choose passive euthanasia for a patient?

2. Is there a difference between active euthanasia for animals and active euthanasia for human beings? Explain.

3. Write a statement of euthanasia that might be considered for legislation.

4. How would you deal with a situation as a nurse in a hospital nursery where orders from the medical staff and family indicate "Do not feed," for a genetically deformed infant?

5. Is passive euthanasia closely related to postponing death by artificial means? Explain.

6. A patient who has recently been diagnosed as having a terminal illness comes to your office with a properly executed Living Will. What procedures will you follow?

CHAPTER 19

DYING AND DEATH

LEARNING OBJECTIVES

Upon successful completion of this chapter, you will:

1. List at least eight generalizations of suffering and dying.
2. Compare short-term and long-term suffering.
3. Describe the importance of medications for dying patients.
4. Identify and explain at least five *psychological* aspects affecting dying patients.
5. Identify and explain at least five *physiological* aspects affecting dying patients.
6. Discuss the stages of dying as defined by Kübler-Ross.
7. Describe hospice for dying patients.
8. Compare the Living Will and the Natural Death Act.
9. Explain the role of physicians and office employees with regard to dying patients.
10. Recall the two legal definitions of death.
11. Discuss the Uniform Anatomical Gift Act.
12. Describe an autopsy and who may authorize one.
13. Explain the role of physicians and office employees with regard to survivors following a death.

INTRODUCTION

There is one thing very certain in life, and that is death. Each of us will die. It will be early for some; late for others. Death may come suddenly with no warning. Death may come slowly, and it may be accompanied by much pain and suffering. In the latter situation, dying becomes a process or a preparation for the final conclusion—death.

SUFFERING IN DYING

Dying and suffering are personal events. No two people will suffer and die alike. To attempt to identify any particular models in suffering and dying is fruitless. None exists. Each person is unique and the life experiences brought to the situation are varied. However, some generalizations can be made.

1. The way persons live is often mirrored in the way they die.
2. Persons with useful "support systems," such as friends, family, and faith in life, may find this support helpful in dying.
3. Experiencing the death of someone close brings the reality of dying into focus.
4. Intellectual preparation for dying, such as writing your will and planning your funeral, may ease the fear of death.
5. Relationships with families and friends will change.
6. Basic personalities usually remain unchanged, but moods may vary radically.
7. Personal goals will be re-evaluated.
8. Pain, suffering, and dependence are feared most by the dying.
9. Dying is not a casual experience.
10. The age of dying persons will, in part, determine their reaction to death.
11. Cultural mores will influence attitudes toward death.

Short-term suffering presents a set of problems different from those of long-term suffering. This can best be seen in the following situation.

A 45-year-old teacher learned in June that chronic myelocytic leukemia accompanied by blastic transformation was destroying her body. The prognosis was poor. Hospitalization and chemotherapy followed, with severe side effects and pain. She died two months later, never returning home.

A 50-year-old electrician was diagnosed as having cancer of the colon. Surgery followed and a permanent colostomy was established. Postoperatively, the patient did well and later returned to work part-time. Within a year cancer metastasized and complications resulted. Consultation with specialists recommended only symptomatic treatment. His pain required massive doses of analgesics to keep him comfortable for the remaining six months. The electrician was unable to return to work but remained home until about six weeks prior to death, when he was again hospitalized.

In a comparison of these two illustrations, time, costs, and dependency are three variables to consider. Obviously, the time of pain and suffering is longer for the electrician than the teacher. The severity, however, cannot be compared. Overall costs are far greater for the electrician than the teacher, but nothing is known of insurance coverage or family resources. Either situation could be a financial burden on survivors. Dependency of these patients upon their friends and family is somewhat different. The teacher had to depend upon someone to take care of any personal matters, which might include job, children, and finances, for approximately two months. The electrician, however, was dependent upon family for physical and nursing care in the home. He also needed someone to take care of personal matters from diagnosis to death, approximately 18 months.

Even the length of time is difficult to establish. Time is relative. Two months and eighteen months may both be considered short-term, when compared to an individual in a state of semiconsciousness for four or five years.

USE OF MEDICATIONS

Medications will be used by the suffering when dying both in the hospital and at home. The greatest difficulty with medications will arise in long-term suffering.

Medications are given for many reasons. They will include analgesics for pain, sedatives for sleep, and specific medications for the particular disease condition. Antidepressants and tranquilizers also may be prescribed. Medications are to be respected for their intended action and the patient's needs.

Problems arise when family members, friends, and even allied health professionals circumvent or question the physician's orders for medications. This is often disastrous for the patient. It is wise for all persons close to the patient to understand the physician's orders and the use of the prescribed medications. Family members should know the reasoning of the physician so any questions arising will not be misunderstood. For example, imagine the fear a spouse feels when the pharmacist says, "Do you know this is a near-lethal dose?" Unless the spouse knows that this amount is needed to keep the pain level of the patient bearable, the spouse may withhold the medication, and may even begin to distrust the physician. It is important to realize that medications may be given in different dosages, frequencies, and combinations for a dying patient than for others. Another problem is that chronic painful diseases are less responsive to analgesics than are other diseases.[1]

PSYCHOLOGICAL ASPECTS OF DYING

Dying patients differ in their psychological experiences. While basic *personalities* remain the same, changes will occur. A person normally calm and loving may have periods of violence and hatred. A happy person may become severely depressed. An individual who is usually accepting of medical fact may totally deny a terminal illness.

Relationships may change. Some individuals are incapable of continuing a close relationship with a person who is dying. Closest friends may become aloof and distant. Some also may fear touching or caressing the dying person. The dying person also can reject any close contact or relationships. The following quotation, words from a dying person, illustrates this controversy. "I am not sure why, but I want to accept, and end up rejecting; I want to love, but often show hostility; I find peace, but am often afraid; I am willing to surrender, but more often seek to control."[2] The opposite also may be true. A stronger bond of friendship can develop, and new friendships will be made, possibly from individuals in similar circumstances. Broken relationships may be healed.

Relationships are important and should be encouraged. They provide strength and support that may not be available through any other source.

The depth of relationships during this time and the degree of acceptance by dying persons may depend on their *self-image*. When a person is ill, is in pain, lives in a deteriorating body, and possibly is unable to perform the activities of daily living, self-image is fragile. When self-image is lacking, hope is lost; dying persons feel useless, may think they are burdens, and will have difficulties accepting help. The psychological effect of a poor self-image may even hasten death.

Dying patients may not be physically able to continue working. If they are sole wage earners, this may present a real financial crisis, especially if the unemployed period extends for a long time. Unemployed patients may be bored, feel useless, may worry, and their self-image suffers.

Personal goals are altered or may even become nonexistent for the dying. Goals such as seeing a child graduate or a grandchild born may be seen as unrealistic to the dying because of the limited time factor. The dying will either give up or strive to live to that event. The total loss of personal goals, no matter how insignificant they may appear, can be devastating to the dying and to persons caring for them. *Indecision* is often a psychological dilemma accompanying the lack of personal goals. It is common for persons close to the dying to recommend goals and help in the decision-making process. This must be done sensitively and realistically.

Communication may become difficult. Aside from any psychological problems, what dying persons are able to understand or hear may depend on what they choose to hear or are ready to understand. Communication may be complicated further if there has not been honesty about the patient's condition. It is possible, of course, for the opposite to be true. Some dying persons express the ability to communicate with greater depth because of the urgency of their circumstances.

An area causing communication difficulties is whether dying patients should be told of their terminal condition. How much information should they be given? Proponents agree that all patients need to be told the medical facts by physicians and treated openly and honestly by all health professionals. They believe informed patients are better able to face death and are less afraid of the truth than are many health professionals. Opponents believe no patients should be told they are dying. Others believe only those patients who give some verbal/nonverbal indication that they want to know should be told. Only patients who can handle the truth should be told. Some patients may refuse to set goals, give up hope, and wait impatiently for death.

Fear is often a traumatic psychological aspect of dying. There is fear of pain, fear of long suffering, fear of losing independence, fear of financial ruin, and fear of death itself. It is important for the patient's fears to be recognized and alleviated, if possible. To recognize the fears requires active and passive listening on the part of all persons close to the dying as well as a willingness on the part of the dying to express their fears.

Much fear can be lessened if persons close to the dying anticipate the fear and provide possible solutions and appropriate resources. Outside help may be sought, if necessary. Social workers, public health nurses, home health aides, clergy, and other health professionals can be valuable resources. Patients' fears should be taken seriously and reference to their unimportance should be avoided.

The psychological aspects of death are difficult because they may not be tangible. They are generally less understood than the physiological aspects of death and quite often left to laypersons rather than professionals. To care for the physical and ignore the psychological is to treat only half the patient.

PHYSIOLOGICAL ASPECTS

Medicine has numerous treatments for some of the physiological problems of suffering and pain experienced in the dying process. Sometimes the treatments are sufficient; other times, they barely address the problem. Untreated or undiagnosed physiological problems may cause or enhance psychological difficulties for dying patients.

It is difficult to separate the psychological from the physiological. For example, pain and suffering, if untreated by therapy or medicinal means, may prove to be a psychological barrier for patients, their families, and health professionals.

Loss of communication skills, such as in the aphasic patient, may be frustrating and unbearable. If patients are *indecisive* or *senile* due to physiological changes, they may not be able to participate in the decision-making process of their terminal illness. Family members may need to assume greater roles in talking for patients and making decisions.

Other common physiological problems encountered include *loss of bodily functions, inability to move or ambulate, inability to eat or drink, inability to tolerate* medications, treatments, light or sound. In the hospital setting, these symptoms may be treated without much difficulty. However, if patients choose to die at home, professional help or training may prove valuable. If patients become severely handicapped physically, they may be reluctant to go anywhere, even to the medical office. Family members may become exhausted caring for them or be unable to administer some of their treatments. The more severe these physiological problems, the more difficulty daily existence becomes.

Physiological difficulties may hinder *sexual identity and involvement.* Dying patients' sexuality may be affected through their love play leading to the sexual response cycle; it may affect endurance necessary for this cycle to occur; or it may affect the desire for physical sexual expression.[3] The physiological and psychological aspects of sexuality are so intertwined that "cause" and "effect" are difficult to determine. A discussion of sexuality and related patients' problems needs to be initiated. If necessary, partners should be considered.

Physiological as well as psychological problems need to be anticipated, diagnosed, and treated. Treating the physiological and psychological aspects of patients enables total patient care.

STAGES OF DYING

Elisabeth Kübler-Ross defines five stages or responses of dying persons. These include *denial, anger, bargaining, depression,* and *acceptance.* There is no set time period for any one stage nor will every dying person go through each and every stage consecutively. Some patients may stay in denial until death, others may manage denial and bargaining and stumble in depression. Still others may move back and forth from one stage to another. There is no set or acceptable pattern. Each dying patient is an individual. However, the stages do offer information on how to relate with patients.

Denial: Patients may deny their terminal illness or go through periods of disbelief. Sometimes it is a result of shock when they are first told. It is common to hear patients say, "This is not happening to me." "I'll go to another physician to see what's wrong." Denial is generally a temporary defense and offers therapeutic meaning to patients. Medical office employees need to listen to patients during this stage. Trying to contradict patients or force them to believe what is happening to them will be to no avail.

Anger: Patients suddenly realize, "It is me. This is happening to me. Why me?" They become "problem patients" and are envious and resentful. Anger may be dispersed in all directions, at people and toward the environment. Rage and temper tantrums can occur. Professionals and family members need to be understanding no matter how angry the patient becomes. Listening to the patient is important to allow patients to vent their own feelings.

Bargaining: During this stage, patients will try to make a deal with their physicians, God, or family, usually for more time or periods of comfort without pain. Patients tend to be more cooperative and congenial. Some common patient responses are, "Please let me see my homeland again." "I'll be so good, if I can just have three pain-free hours." "Dear God, I'll never . . . if you make me well." Medical office employees need to listen to dying patients' requests, but not become a party to the bargain. Some bargaining may be associated with guilt, and any indication of this should be mentioned to the physician. Bargaining can have a positive affect. It may give the patient the hope and stamina to reach a desired goal.

Depression: The dying patient's body is deteriorating, sometimes rapidly, financial burdens are increasing, pain is unbearable and relationships severed. All can lead to depression. They are losing everything and everyone they love. It may be a time of tears, and crying may allow relief. Professionals who are happy, loud, and reassuring will not provide much help to depressed patients. Patients may need to express their sorrow to someone, or merely have someone close. There may be little need for words in this stage.

Acceptance: The final but perhaps not a lasting stage is when patients are accepting of their fate. They usually are tired, weak, and able to sleep. They are not necessarily happy, rather at peace. Professionals need to be aware patients may prefer to be left alone, not bothered with world events or family problems. Family members usually require more help, understanding, and support than patients. Touching and the use of silence may prove useful.

HOSPICE

Hospice is a French word meaning host. Webster defines it as a lodging for travelers or young persons, especially when maintained by a religious order. The term was later used to describe lodging for dying persons. The first hospice, Saint Christopher's, was formed by Dr. Cecily Saunders in London in 1965. Since then the hospice concept has moved throughout the United States.

Hospices provide care of the terminally ill at home, in a hospital, or a special facility. The main objective of that care is to make patients comfortable, "at home," and close to family. Treatments such as CPR, intravenous therapy, nasogastric tubes, and antibiotics are discouraged. Treatments are given in light of the patient's personal and social circumstances.

The hospice staff attempts to create a positive atmosphere. Death is seen as "all right." A balance is kept between human needs and medical needs. Children are encouraged to be in the hospice as a reminder that life is an ongoing process.[4] Patients might share a cup of tea with staff and each other rather than receiving an intravenous solution during their last hours.

Advantages the hospice offers include staff members who are experienced and want to care for the dying. Its services are provided only to the dying, and death is managed with dignity. The dying patient is not isolated behind curtains, but rather is surrounded by others. An empty bed remains empty for at least 24 hours to allow adjustment by everyone. Another advantage is that the survivors are helped to deal with the death. If the hospice care is at home, patients are in familiar surroundings, have their favorite food, and are close to loved ones.

Disadvantages of the hospice exist. One problem is "Can family members, with hospice's help, handle the care at home?" It may be too much, physically and emotionally. Also, what about dying patients? Are they comfortable with the kind of care they receive in the hospice? Do they need or want more? Are they comfortable in dealing with death? We may be conditioned to expect dying patients to be in hospitals, not homes. One research study indicated that 80 percent of relatives preferred to have their terminally ill loved ones die in the hospital, while 80 percent of dying persons said they preferred to die at home.[5]

LIVING WILL

A living will is a document made by a living person, voluntarily, stating what is to be done in the event of a terminal illness, especially when comatose or incompetent. It generally means certain heroic or extraordinary measures are prohibited. A living will also may address a desire to die at home and/or donate organs.

It is generally agreed that for the living will to be valid, legislation is required. Only ten states have living will statutes,[6]* and many of these create legal havoc. One statute says "life shall not be prolonged beyond the point of meaningful existence."[7] What is meaningful? Meaningful to whom?

To improve the living will's effectiveness, Annas, Glantz, and Katz[8] make two suggestions: 1) have patients appoint representatives to speak on their behalf, and 2) make the living will binding on its caretakers. Further precautions may include making sure the document is consistent with state law, is readily available to all possible caregivers and family members, can-

---

*California, Idaho, Nevada, Texas, Oregon, Arkansas, New Mexico, North Carolina, Washington, Kansas.

not be misinterpreted, and for states to provide punishment for deviations from the stated will.

NATURAL DEATH ACT

Some states have attempted to answer the legal imperfections of the living will by adopting a Natural Death Act. California was the first state to pass legislation and Washington soon followed. Most critics agree that the California act is "cumbersome, confusing and likely to create more problems than it solves."[9] Two flaws are that, for the document to be binding, it must be signed 14 days or more after a terminal illness has been diagnosed. Qualified witnesses are so restricted it would be difficult to find one. Washington's Natural Death Act is relatively new and untried by the courts. Time will tell its effectiveness.

Even though living wills and Natural Death Acts are confusing and pose legal questions, they do govern the actions of health care providers, and knowledge of these statutes is vital.

ROLE OF PHYSICIAN AND OFFICE EMPLOYEE

Terminally ill patients have special needs. Their reactions in the dying process are expressed in their various stages or responses. No matter how "good" or "bad" they present themselves, medical office employees need to assess where patients are and react openly to them.

One of the best ways to begin reacting to the dying patient is to take a good, hard look at your own attitude toward pain, suffering, and dying. How can you be especially sensitive to these patients without being obvious? Will you be able to respond to the patients' total needs rather than merely their medical needs? Can you be comfortable when patients cry, when patients laugh, when they joke about their condition?

Health care professionals need to be able to talk without fear or anxiety to provide information as well as to listen to dying patients. For example, a medical office employee may be asked, "Will I get addicted to these narcotics?" If the employee's thoughts are, "The doctor never should have given you anything so powerful," this attitude will be sensed by the patient verbally and/or nonverbally.

Dying patients may exhibit negative or distasteful behaviors in the office. How will you handle it? Will you take it personally? Will you react negatively? Ignore it?

Patients may ask questions with hidden meaning or be truly blunt. Are you aware of nonverbal clues from patients? How will you react? What if you do not know any answers?

Dying patients may develop gross physical deformities or radically altered physical appearances. Will you be able to manage? If so, how?

Family and friends will require your attention, too. What will you do when you "reach the end of *your* rope" and become too emotionally involved?

Patient referrals may be made to counselors, pastors, attorneys, social workers, and hospice organizations. Do not fool yourself that you can be all things to all people. Medical office employees need to feel free to refer.

LEGAL DEFINITIONS OF DEATH

In previous years, one of the most widely accepted definitions of death was from Black's Law Dictionary:[10]

The cessation of life; the ceasing to exist; defined by physicians as a total stoppage of the circulation of the blood, and a cessation of the animal and vital functions consequent thereon, such as respiration, pulsation, etc. . . .

Today with medical advances, resuscitative devices, increased complexities of life, and organ transplants, Black's definition of death is insufficient. Death is a continuum and different parts of the body die at different times. The heart may stop before or after the patient dies. For example, in a heart attack victim, the heart stops beating but the patient does not die immediately. It takes three to four minutes before there is irreparable brain death. At this point, the patient is dead. Once the brain dies, there is no need for the other body organs, and they die at various intervals.[11]

The concept of brain death was presented by the Harvard Ad-Hoc Committee, chaired by Henry Beecher. The criteria are simple:

A patient in this state appears to be in deep coma. The condition can be satisfactorily diagnosed by the following points: 1) Unreceptivity and unresponsivity, 2) no movements/breathing, 3) no reflexes and 4) flat electroencephalogram (EEG). Each of the above tests shall be repeated at least 24 hours later with no change. This definition of brain death does not cover cases such as Karen Ann Quinlan, who is in a "persistent vegetative state" or people who are in comas but do not meet other accepted criteria. Most agree that the brain-death concept is truly in accord with modern medical, moral, and ethical thinking.

UNIFORM ANATOMICAL GIFT ACT

This new definition—of brain death—was essential especially in the area of organ transplants. Under the old definition, a surgeon removing a vital organ from a body still breathing and pulsating could technically be guilty of homicide. Many states, therefore, have adopted legislation making brain death legal.

All fifty states have some form of the Uniform Anatomical Gift Act. Persons 18 years or older and of sound mind may make a gift of all or any part of their body to the following persons for the following purposes:

1. To any hospital, surgeon, or physician for medical or dental education, research, advancement of medical or dental science, therapy, or transplantation.
2. To any accredited medical or dental school, college, or university for education, research, advancement of medical or dental science, or therapy.
3. To any bank or storage facility, for medical or dental education, research, advancement of medical or dental science, therapy, or transplantation.
4. To any specified individual for therapy or transplantation needed by him.

The gift may be made by a provision in a will or by signing, in the presence of two witnesses, a card. The card is generally carried with the person at all times.[13]

Persons may place conditions on their organ donation. If a relative(s) opposes the donation, most physicians and hospitals would not insist on the transplant. Donors are carefully screened before their body parts are used. The physician and hospital may be found negligent and so they must have strict standards for donor screening.

AUTOPSY

An autopsy is an examination of a dead body to determine the cause of death. Statutes generally state who can authorize an autopsy. Coroners or medical examiners may give such authorization. Others include, in order of priority:

1. surviving spouse.
2. any child of the deceased who is 18 years of age or older
3. any one of the parents of the deceased
4. any adult brother or sister of the deceased.

Autopsies may be complete or partial. In other words, a pathologist may perform an autopsy on the entire body, and examine every part and organ, or merely do an autopsy of the thoracic cavity or the brain. The extremities rarely are involved unless indicated by trauma, prior surgical procedure, or vessel involvement. No part(s) of the body can be retained for any reason, without consent from the family. If the autopsy is done properly and in a professional manner, the body can be viewed by survivors and/or at a funeral.

There are circumstances that require an autopsy. (Refer to Chapter 5, Public Duties, for further information.) Autopsies certainly offer valuable information for medical science and research. It is important for survivors to understand knowledge gained from an autopsy may prevent another person from suffering similar circumstances.

ROLE OF THE PHYSICIAN AND MEDICAL OFFICE EMPLOYEE

After the patient has died, physicians and employees need to turn their focus to survivors. In telling survivors of the death, it is best to be honest and caring. It is a shocking and painful time for survivors and they will need your utmost attention. Try to provide whatever support they need and remain with them until some family or close friends can come.

Some time during the grieving process, survivors may call or come to your office for information or assistance. If you are unable to answer their questions or meet their needs, refer them to someone who can. Funeral directors and the clergy offer valuable help in planning the funeral, answering questions about the human remains or helping survivors through the grieving process. Organizations such as Compassionate Friends (parents who have lost a child) and widow-widowers can be recommended, if appropriate.

Communication with survivors may be especially difficult for office employees. You may be afraid to say dead and died. *Dead Is a Four Letter Word* (a title of a book by Lynn Melby) tells us much about our feelings of death. Once we explore our attitudes and feelings on death, we can be more useful to survivors.

Children and death pose sensitive situations. Death of a child is a profound emotional experience for everyone, especially family. Explaining death to a child also is difficult. The age and maturity of children need to be taken into consideration. Children deserve the same honesty as an adult and need to be told that sorrow is very acceptable and that it is okay to cry. Reassure children that death is in no way their fault. Using a phrase such as, "God took your Daddy away" may cause the child to blame God. Follow the lead of children in their questions. It is important to tell children that you do not have all the answers. Memories should be cherished and encouraged. Children require the same ritual and sorrow that other family members go through.[14]

Volumes of materials have been written in the past decade on the subject of dying and death. The information in this chapter only highlights the areas that seem most appropriate for the medical office. There are some resources, however, that we would like to recommend for your personal reading as they have been especially helpful. They are as follows:

Alsop, S.: *Stay of Execution.* J.B. Lippincott Company, 1973

Ashbrook, J. B.: *Responding to Human Pain.* Judson Press, Valley Forge, PA 19481, 1975

Barnard, C.: *Good Life, Good Death, A Doctor's Case for Euthanasia and Suicide.* Prentice-Hall, Inc., Englewood Cliffs, New Jersey, 1980.

Flint, C.R.: *Grief's Slow Wisdom.* Droke House, Publishers, Anderson, South Carolina; Distributed by Grossett and Dunlap, 51 Madison Avenue, New York.

Griffith, W. H.: *Confronting Death, Help from the Minister, Physician, Funeral Director and Lawyer.* Judson Press, Valley Forge, PA 19481, 1977.

Grollman, E.A.: *Explaining Death to Children.* Beacon Press, Boston, 1972.

Hayes, D.M.: *Between Doctor and Patient.* Judson Press, Valley Forge, PA 19481, 1977.

Kübler-Ross, E.: *On Death and Dying.* The Macmillan Company, New York, 1972.

Lear, M.W.: *Heartsounds.* Pocket Books, a Simon & Schuster Division of Gulf & Western Corporation, New York, 1980.

Melby, L.L.: *Dead Is a Four Letter Word.* Dabney Publishing, 1826 North 45, Seattle, WA 98103, 1975.

Simonton, O.C.: *Getting Well Again.* Stephanie Matthews-Simonton, James L. Creighton, Bantam Books, Inc., New York, 1980.

Smith, J.K.: *Free Fall.* Judson Press, Valley Forge, PA 19481, 1975.

REFERENCES

1. HAYES, DM: *Between Doctor and Patient.* Judson, Valley Forge, 1977, p 136.
2. SMITH, JK: *Free Fall.* Judson, Valley Forge, 1975, p 7.
3. WERNER-BELAND, JA: *Grief Responses to Long-Term Illness and Disability.* Reston, Reston, VA, 1980, p 68.
4. GORDON, A: *A Touch of Wonder.* Guideposts Associates, Carmel, NY, p 243.
5. BARNARD, C: *Good Life, Good Death.* Prentice-Hall, Englewood Cliffs, NJ, 1980, p 21.
6. ANNAS, GJ, GLANTZ, LH AND KATZ, BF: *The Rights of Doctors, Nurses and Allied Health Professionals.* Avon Books, New York, NY, 1981, p 221.
7. *Death with dignity.* The International Journal of Medicine and Law 1:2, Haifa, Israel, 1979, p 182.
8. ANNAS, p 221.
9. *Death with dignity,* p 182.
10. BLACK, HC: *Black's Law Dictionary,* ed 4. West, St Paul, Minnesota, 1951, p 488.
11. BARNARD, pp 6-7.
12. YEZZI, R: *Medical Ethics.* Holt, Rinehart and Winston, New York, 1980, p 113.
13. ANNAS, p 228.
14. MELBY, L: *Dead Is a Four Letter Word.* Dabney, Seattle, 1975, pp 15-20.

DISCUSSION QUESTIONS

1. Are there any generalizations on death that you might add to the authors'? Any you might delete? Which ones most likely would describe you?

2. Describe some problems faced by family members in a long-term illness.

3. Does the allocation of scarce medical resources influence the care given to someone who is dying?

4. List Kübler-Ross's five stages of dying and give an example of each.

5. A patient leaves the medical office and says to the receptionist, "I know I am dying. You people are lying to me." What is your response?

6. Would you prefer to die in a hospice or a hospital?

7. A patient asks, "How do I make out a Living Will?" What resources can you recommend?

8. If your community hospital does not have an electroencephalograph, how will death be determined?

9. How can you donate your organs?

10. Under what circumstances might physicians decide not to tell patients they are dying?

11. What considerations are taken into account when telling a child about death?

12. Why might an autopsy be helpful? Why might one be refused?

13. What have you done to prepare for your own death? Do you have a will? Have you planned for your family? Have you made any decisions that should be shared with legal counsel and/or physicians?

CHAPTER **20**

HAVE A CARE!

LEARNING OBJECTIVES

Upon successful completion of this chapter, you will:

1. Cry.
2. Laugh.
3. Experience a patient's dilemma in the medical office.
4. Become a little more human.

I am a patient with an appointment to see your physician at 10:30 today. It is early December.

I hurt, I can't function at home, I can't function at work. The pain in my back is so bad I can't lift my five-month-old infant. It hurts to shower and turn the steering wheel of the car. I have to go to bed before my husband and then I can't move—the spasms are terrifying. They wake me.

I am so tired. I have no energy. I'm not really afraid. I trust the doctor; I know he'll find out what is wrong—fix it—and I'll be back to normal.

I'm taking time from work to be here. It is inconvenient, but I can do it. No one will do my job while I'm gone; it will wait for my return. It has to be done. I expect action today, though. I don't want sympathy.

I'm glad I don't have to wait long in your office. The pain is a little less; the psychological release from knowing I'll soon be better is addicting. But I put up a front, too. I can't cry or tell the doctor how bad it really is. The office greeting is cheerful, but I could use some help with my clothes. I can hardly get them off. The bra is terrible, and the pantyhose are worse.

Your physician is quiet, professional, and concerned. I feel better just seeing him. His smile is warm. I can tell he cares. The examination is not too difficult. He finally says, "It looks serious. We have to run a lot of tests. It is going to take time to get to the bottom of this." Lab tests and x-rays are ordered. Any physical activity is allowed *until* it causes pain. I don't tell him how hard that will be. He tells me to bring my husband with me the next visit. I'm instructed to get dressed and go to the lab. The awful bra and pantyhose again—and it hurts to tie my shoes.

The atmosphere is sterile in the lab—cool and "too" professional. My mind is racing while I wait. I'm in torment. "What is it? What about my baby? Will I be able to take care of her? I've waited 36 years for her. Am I going to be a burden?"

The lab technician withdraws the blood and I give the lab a urine specimen. The awful pantyhose again! "Collect a 24-hour urine." They hand me this weird antifreeze-like container with an opening like a vinegar bottle. It is white and has large black letters, "For 24° Urine Only." I also am told to collect some feces. I'm handed three unfolded cardboard containers and some tiny spatulas. No instructions. I can leave—with the antifreeze container and all!

As I leave, I wonder, how long do I wait? When will I know? I'm exhausted. I want to get home and see my husband. I need to talk to someone. Oh, the pain is bad. I hurt.

*   *   *

A telephone call a week later from your physician tells me the progress of the tests, but no indication of a diagnosis. He is very general in his conversation.

Christmas is a blur. There is no change in my condition. Questions from family and friends are no help. They don't understand. Neither do I. I hide my true feelings.

*   *   *

I'm back in your office a few weeks later with my husband. He had to take time from work. The receptionist seems surprised that my husband is with me. I wonder if she thinks I can't handle this. Well, I can't!

The consultation is hard. Your physician is open and honest. He tells us that there is a bone disease that is rampant—it is a metabolic bone disorder. I hear him tell my husband that I can have no physical activity. I must take off work. I cannot drive. To fall would be disastrous. My bones are like a loaf of bread. "You know what a loaf of bread is like when it is smashed." I cannot lift anything—even my baby. I'm not supposed to bend over. My husband asks, "Should we have outside help come into the home?" The doctor says, "Yes." I immediately think about the cost. The doctor tells me what kind of medications I'll be taking. But the final blow is his words that there is something else wrong. He hopes more tests will reveal what.

*   *   *

A month passes. I'm having such a hard time having someone do *my* work. I find a replacement at my job. I don't ask for help easily. It is so hard to be inactive. I can't get my own groceries. I'm terrified of falling. I can't vacuum my floors. I can't lift my baby to change her. If she cries, I can't pick her up. Having someone else do those things I'm supposed to do is terrible. And when no one is looking, I do lift her. I do carry her. And I do damage my body. This creates conflict with my husband. Life is not good.

During this time, there are more tests and more referrals. More doctors. I feel like a "nothing." I feel inhuman. The worst tests are the intestinal or small bowel biopsies. Your physician tells me that they put a tube in my mouth, pass it through to the small intestine. It is painless and won't take very long.

My husband takes me to the test and is told I'll be finished in about 1 1/2 hours. They will call him. In the exam room, I'm partially disrobed and I put on a 3/4 length gown that opens down the back. I can keep my slacks and shoes on. The gastroenterologist passed the tube through my mouth into my stomach. There is no pain, but it is awful. I gag over and over again. I must try not to. I tell myself to breathe slowly; concentrate on not vomiting. When the gastroenterologist finishes, the LPN says, "Let's go to x-ray."

To my horror, she hands me a box of tissues and an emesis basin, drapes my coat over my shoulders, takes my elbow, and says, "Be careful not to fall." I bite on the tube in my mouth and try to stabilize it with my free hand as we walk through a large, crowded reception area, out the front door, across two office parking lots covered with early morning frost. Still in disbelief, we walk into the lowest floor of a multiple-office building where the x-ray receptionist tells us the radiologist is still at the hospital making rounds. I snarl through my teeth, "Get that doctor here *now*."

In the x-ray waiting area I sit for 30 minutes, still trying not to gag. The tears come, first haltingly, then freely. The saliva flows from my mouth and nose. I'm finally able to get hold of myself. I stop crying. I don't want to ruin the test. Finally the doctor appears. He looks at me; in my revulsion at the situation and him, I whisper, "You son-of-a_____!" His response is, "What's wrong with you?" How can I tell him? I still have the tube in my mouth. He checks the placement of the tube in the small intestine several different times. When he verifies that it is in place, he calls another LPN to take me back. Over the same route. I pray to God no one recognizes me. I am in a state of shock about my circumstances.

Upon returning, the biopsy is taken. The doctor pulls the tube; I sigh with relief. In a few minutes, he turns to me and says, "We didn't get it." The instrument to snatch a piece of the intestinal wall didn't grab properly. The same process must be done again. The tube goes back in—across the parking lots—check the tube—back across the parking lots. This time, the biopsy is successful!

My husband is trying to call the office—wondering what has happened. They tell him only that there is a problem. He's not allowed to speak to anyone else. Four and one-half hours later, they call to tell him I'm finished.

*   *   *

Months have passed. I'm now living with the metabolic bone disorder, and an intestinal malabsorption problem. Both are improving. I am back to work. My activities are somewhat limited, with lifting still a problem. It is hard not to lift and "rough" play with my daughter, but I no longer need help at home. I must take much medication, some of it experimental, and I'm four inches shorter, but the prognosis is good.

I enjoy life. I enjoy my work. My family gives me strength. I've loved being an author of this book. Why do I share this with you when I've never told anyone other than my family?

The reason is that the authors want to leave with you some impressions on the importance of caring.

Take from it what you may. Please remember to be loving, to be gracious, to be human, to be able to put yourself in the place of your patients. Consider circumstances of your patients, not just in your offices, but in all facets of their lives.

DISCUSSION QUESTIONS

1. Was any health professional a "listener" for this patient?
2. What kind of nonverbal messages did the patient send?

3. What positive forms of conduct and courtesy were shown to the patient?

4. What negative forms of conduct and courtesy were shown to the patient?

5. What could you have done as a receptionist, as a nurse, as a lab technician, as a medical assistant, and as a physician?

EPILOGUE

This book has been written for you. You who are employed in a medical office; you who are students in medical assisting or other allied health programs in schools; you who are physicians spending the major portion of your working day in your office treating patients.

We have cared for your patients at home; we have worked in your offices and hospitals; we have taught in your classes; we have been your patients. We know the great responsibility you carry as employees; we delight in your excitement about preparing yourself to work for physicians; we appreciate your role as physicians and business managers of the medical office.

We have not tried to be your legal counsel; we have not attempted to know all your state's statutes; we have not wanted to be your conscience in the complex world of bioethics.

We hope we have been your guide; we hope we have stimulated your interest in the law; we hope we have aroused your compassion and empathy for any person struggling for answers in any of the issues in bioethics; we hope you have a practical text for the classroom; we hope you have a handbook for quick reference in the medical office; we hope you buy a hundred thousand copies.

We have laughed; we have cried; we have driven 4,000 miles from Seattle to Bremerton and vice versa—a distance of only 50 miles; we have sweated; we have written, revised, rewritten, and typed; we have sought legal advice; we have eaten hundreds of lemon drops; we have learned; we have expanded our horizons; we have given birth to a book; and a strong bond of love and friendship has developed.

BUT NOW IT IS YOURS!

INDEX